Praise for *Your Body Will Show You the Way*

"This delicious book teaches you how to listen and make sense of what your body is saying, and how to respond creatively. You're going to love Ellen Meredith's new energy medicine techniques to support awakening and change. I really believe that your life will be empowered and strengthened forever when you feel the confidence to communicate with your own body and allow your energies to guide you into better health and more joy and vitality — plus, you will have these tools for a lifetime. I am going to shout about this book from the rooftops! Superb!"

— **Donna Eden**, bestselling author of *Energy Medicine*

"Ellen will help you develop new ways of understanding and communicating with your body. You'll learn to see with fresh eyes the situations in your life that have previously kept you stuck.... Ellen invites us to nothing less than a rebirth of ourselves, understanding the possibilities we have to shift and change and grow into a future we truly desire. These simple ideas are magnificent in their scope and can lead to a new reality within your physical body and your life."

— from the foreword by **Lauren Walker**, creator of Energy Medicine Yoga and bestselling author of *The Energy to Heal*

"*Your Body Will Show You the Way* is the title and promise of Ellen Meredith's new book, and Ellen certainly does show us the way. She breaks boundaries, gets us thinking, inspires, motivates, and guides us in new ways of self-care, tapping into ancient wisdom that helps us deal with modern life and its challenges. This innovative book is without doubt a must-read!"

— **Madison King**, mentor, teacher, and author of *Everyday Energy*

"I couldn't wait to get my hands on this book! So often we block ourselves from our own healing abilities. This book will help you discover how to both listen and respond to your body so you can begin to heal, grow, and thrive both inside and out. The techniques shared are clear and easy to follow, and Ellen Meredith's fun-loving style of writing makes this book easy to digest. A must-read for anyone interested in learning more about the amazing power of bodily wisdom."

— **Sherianna Boyle,**
135 Self-Guided Practices to

"If you are sensitive by nature and want to develop a deeper relationship with your body and your inner strength, *Your Body Will Show You the Way* works as a brilliant and loving map. Ellen Meredith's book also includes powerfully vulnerable storytelling, which makes it so relatable. Full of insights and exercises, this book will help you bridge spirit, earth, and your body in a loving, concise, and very timely way."

— **Lee Harris**, author of *Energy Speaks*

"*Your Body Will Show You the Way* is a brilliant guide to resolving our issues at every level. Ellen Meredith has given us comprehensive, practical, and effective tools for internal dialogue, much needed as we deal with the overwhelming stresses of our time. Thank you!"

— **Devi Stern**, advanced Eden Method practitioner and author of *Energy Healing with the Kabbalah*

"Ellen Meredith's *Your Body Will Show You the Way* is an essential guidebook for navigating these turbulent times of change, both personally and collectively. Come home to yourself through these easy-to-follow, transformational practices as you add your light to the world. Start today to live with more grace, ease, and joy! I highly recommend it!"

— **Karen R. Onofrio, MD**, certified Eden Method practitioner

"Once again Ellen Meredith takes us on a deeper, 'inside' journey to unlock our body's own natural healing abilities. Gently guiding us and holding a safe, energetic space, she offers both emotional support and encouragement as she reassures us, 'your body will show you the way.' I encourage you to make a radical change and join Ellen in taking the next step on your inner healing journey to *be well within*."

— **Dr. Melanie Smith**, doctor of Oriental medicine, advanced energy medicine practitioner, teacher, and author of the *Energy Medicine for Healthy Living* and *Tap Into Your Vagus Nerve's Healing Power* online series

Your Body Will Show You the Way

BOOKS AND AUDIO BY ELLEN MEREDITH

Listening In: Dialogues with the Wiser Self

In Search of Radiance: Learning to Stand with Your Wiser Self (audio)

The Language Your Body Speaks: Self-Healing with Energy Medicine

BOOKS PUBLISHED AS ELLEN M. ILFELD

Learning Comes to Life: An Active Learning Program for Teens

Good Beginnings: Parenting in the Early Years, coauthored with J.L. Evans

Early Childhood Counts: A Programming Guide on Early Childhood Care for Development, coauthored with J.L. Evans and R.G. Myers

Your Body Will Show You the Way

Energy Medicine for Personal and Global Change

Ellen Meredith

Foreword by Lauren Walker

New World Library
Novato, California

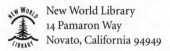

New World Library
14 Pamaron Way
Novato, California 94949

Text design by Tona Pearce Myers

Library of Congress Cataloging-in-Publication Data

Names: Meredith, Ellen, date, author.
Title: Your body will show you the way : energy medicine for personal and global change
    / Ellen Meredith.
Description: Novato, California : New World Library, [2022] | Includes bibliographical
    references and index. | Summary: "A discussion of the principles of energy healing,
    a theory of medicine that views disease as the result of energy imbalances in the
    human body. Includes guided meditations, energy exercises, and stories that illustrate
    key concepts"-- Provided by publisher.
Identifiers: LCCN 2022020300 (print) | LCCN 2022020301 (ebook) | ISBN 9781608688227
    (paperback) | ISBN 9781608688234 (epub)
Subjects: LCSH: Energy medicine. | Mind and body therapies.
Classification: LCC RZ421 .M47 2022 (print) | LCC RZ421 (ebook) | DDC 616.89--dc23/
    eng/20220603
LC record available at https://lccn.loc.gov/2022020300
LC ebook record available at https://lccn.loc.gov/2022020301

First printing, September 2022
ISBN 978-1-60868-822-7
Ebook ISBN 978-1-60868-823-4
Printed in Canada on 100% postconsumer-waste recycled paper

New World Library is proud to be a Gold Certified Environmentally Responsible
Publisher. Publisher certification awarded by Green Press Initiative.

10   9   8   7   6   5   4   3   2   1

To Judith Evans, soul mate,
who held a space and grounded me to write this book…

To Donna Eden, sistah-from-another-mother,
who held a space for me to fly…

Contents

Foreword

It feels like the whole world is teetering on a precipice right now, where our very survival as a species is at stake. Instead of gently walking back from the cliff's edge, we continue to fight about all our problems from opposite sides of a gasping divide. We're like polarized ends of a twirling baton, held apart by a rigid line. This mimics the opposites we feel in so many places in our own bodies and minds. We ping between happy and sad, manic and tired, angry and inspired, productive and frustrated. To mitigate this, many people talk about meeting in the middle — that we should come together in the center from our positions on the poles.

But what if we did something different? Instead of meeting in the middle at some arbitrary point on some arbitrary line, what if instead we allowed ourselves to expand spherically? Take any point of contention and unfold it into a sphere — like the shape created by that spinning baton — not spinning over the cliff, but spinning in a skillful hand. That sphere can encapsulate all of a situation, or all of us together. Not together by making us the same — like dissolving a cup of salt in a cooking pot. But together like a delicious stew — all our differences flavoring the whole. What if we were together in a world of shared understanding, shared differences, a shared desire for safety, love, nourishment, expression?

Perhaps our frustrations about the state of the world and the state of our own health are giving us valuable information that we simply don't understand yet, because it is part of a bigger picture: the picture in the sphere, not the picture in the point. What if we started to look at our desires for personal and global transformation from this new vantage point? Not teetering on the edge, not stuck in the middle, not polarized at the extreme, but encompassing the whole.

That is the vision and the gift that Ellen Meredith shares with us in her new book, *Your Body Will Show You the Way: Energy Medicine for Personal and Global Change.*

I have known Ellen for many years, having studied with her in Donna Eden's school Innersource to learn the inner dynamics of energy healing. As a testament to the power of our shared lineage with Donna (the grandmother energy teacher), Ellen and I have both taken Donna's work and morphed it and translated it through our own lenses and experiences, as many of her students have. I created and wrote three books on Energy Medicine Yoga. And though I studied alongside Ellen for years, I did not know she had her own hidden inner gifts that led her to Donna. She is a magical and talented healer and teacher in her own right. When *The Language Your Body Speaks*, her first book on the power of energy medicine and healing, came out, I was wowed and inspired. And now, in this new book, I am honored to preface her well-tuned gift to you as a seeker of health and wholeness.

Ellen's vision of this new, whole and healed reality manifests in the creation and telling of a new story. The power of this book lies in how skillfully Ellen leads us on the journey of what this new reality might look like and how we might get there.

Nothing less than re-creating our current worldview is called for. The outdated and incorrect vision of ourselves as purely physical beings held hostage by the polar opposites that dominate critical thinking in areas like health care, education, and politics — really every part of our lives and shared experiences — is primed for a change.

To create something new from the pieces of the old is linked to one of my favorite things to do, and that is to *recreate*. Specifically meaning to play, relax, reinvent, and expand into joy and fun. Doing something again and again — like skiing or walking the beach or playing tennis or sitting by a creek — is how we might currently think about recreation. But what if we could *re-create* our worldview — making it better, evolving it, expanding it, and enjoying it? What a fun and different way to look at the world!

I kept dipping into and out of this book, first in the mind of the writer, then in the mind of the student just drinking up knowledge, wisdom, and yes, *stories*. Stories are what we yearn for. They're what give us connection and a deeper meaning in our lives. Stories are how we explain ourselves to ourselves to make sense of the world around us. And stories are what change the narrative.

The stories Ellen shares of her clients are powerful and resonant — people's struggles, challenges, resistances, hopes. Then she steps up to each person, and the magic begins. She leads us through what her energy guides teach her in real time, and then she teaches us how to find those same energies in ourselves, complete with our own personal awareness and transformations.

We're invited right into this wonderfully woven work to re-create our *own* story.

Ellen will help you develop new ways of understanding and communicating with your body. You'll learn to see with fresh eyes the situations in your life that have previously kept you stuck. You'll learn how to reframe your experiences to give you a different perspective. You'll learn how to feel your situation from the inside instead of thinking about it from the outside, and you will gain a whole new experience of simple concepts like grounding and expanding.

Pick up your quill or your paint brush, or your song or your dance, to create and recreate and create again. Ellen guides you to tease apart your difficulties and challenges and understand them in a new way so you can expand into the beautifully shining mosaic of your life; to decrease resistance and discover peace and intimacy with your body and energies; to find healing where healing is possible, and acceptance and calmness in any situation. And from this, she invites you to learn what your body's energies are telling you and how, together with those energies, you can co-create a new, healthier and more easeful reality. A better story.

The teachings here are deceptively simple and fun. In fact, you can do these practices with your whole family; children especially will love the creativity and imagination and engagement. And doing it together with your loved ones and giving the next generation these powerful tools is the perfect way to incorporate this new way of looking at the world.

Ellen invites us to nothing less than a rebirth of ourselves, understanding the possibilities we have to shift and change and grow into a future we truly desire. These simple ideas are magnificent in their scope and can lead to a new reality within your physical body and your life. But Ellen doesn't stop there. She continually draws the parallels between our limited thinking of our own lives and health, and the way we've limited healing in the world as a whole. And she helps us see that we can apply the principles of individual healing to collective and global health. She is offering us a massive paradigm shift.

It is a shift we desperately need right now.

It is a shift we are well poised and positioned to make.

And Ellen's book is one of the best guides to help take us there.

Lauren Walker,
creator of Energy Medicine Yoga
and bestselling author of *The Energy to Heal*

ᖉ Introduction ᖆ

Inner Guidance

It's one of those days when the apparent craziness of the world has gotten to me: my mind has fogged, and I feel exhausted; my gut, head, and muscles ache; my emotions are building up steam, like a pressure cooker. I hear myself start to panic: "Oh no, oh no, what's wrong, what's going on? Am I getting sick?"

If I can stop, hunker down for a moment, and ask, "What do I need right now?," I hear, *Use your hands to cradle your face.*

Then: *Breathe in on a count of three and out on a count of five.*

Then: *Just connect — use your hands to hook up your head and heart, your heart and gut, your front and back, your two feet, et cetera.*

Then I see an image of a spiderweb that has been ravaged by a careless hand. I pull at the threads and rebuild the web, strand by strand.

When I stop to listen and follow the guidance of this awareness inside me step by step, it shifts the logjam of my mind, body, and spirit. The panic lifts, and within a short time, I can see how to proceed with more grace and sanity.

Sometimes the instructions are quite specific. I'm shown a posture to take or a gesture that would help. Other times I'm told something cryptic

I need to unpack and figure out: *Move your headquarters to your solar plexus and think from there.* Or I hear something generic: *Come home. Show up for yourself.* Sometimes I get nothing — no images, no words, no thoughts — and I have to accept the emptiness as my guide.

Tuning to inner guidance was not my initial instinct or what I was programmed to do in this life. I grew up in a family that loved to intellectualize, make theories, talk about grand and far-flung ideas; they tended to ignore the body as an inconvenience. I wasn't taught to respect this instrument, and as a result, I grew increasingly sicker as my physical systems broke down and I had no idea what to do to restore them.

After years of suffering from blood sugar crashes caused by the stress of not knowing how to nourish myself; migraines triggered by competition between my brain and body; and energy rushes and crashes set in motion by a system that revved and strained its engine each time I could not get into gear, I finally understood that my symptoms were a communication and that I needed to show up and participate in the conversation!

I had spent thousands of dollars on tests and treatments, supplements, special diets, healing plans, and trying one recommended road to recovery after another before I finally understood that other people couldn't heal me. The medications and supplements could not heal me. And not even following the recipes for wellness — telling me what ideal diet, sleep habit, exercise, spiritual practice, belief patterning, or lifestyle I should follow — did the trick.

The trick was that I needed to show up, learn how this body, mind, and spirit might best collaborate, and discover what it means for my unique self to get well and flourish.

My body knew how to heal, but I needed to learn how to stop damaging it faster than it could mend and to stop throwing chemical, nutritional, and behavioral "solutions" at it from outside, so I could grow well from the inside out.

Whenever I come home to my body and let the built-in inner guidance system show me what is needed, right now, it changes my world.

☙ • ❧

The suggestions my body guidance gave me were all a form of energy medicine: tools that could shift my body's function and communications energetically, just as pills are designed to shift the body's functions chemically.

I can't pretend that everything I've learned about energy medicine arose solely from dialogue with my body. In my early twenties I was sitting at my typewriter, waiting for inspiration to write a poem or story. Instead, I realized I was seeing a kind of ticker tape in my head, like they used in the old stock market. Only there were letters on the tape instead of numbers. I wrote them down as the text scrolled through my inner screen and then was rather stunned to read this message:

> You have asked to know us, and so we are here. We have been with you for a very long time, and now you are ready to come stand with us. We will work with you. Let your Wiser Self which observes continue the writing at night, and we will come through with a few lines. Simply don't block the connection. Past awareness of us is imminent. Someone will give you a plant to water; be aware of the plant processes of growth. Surely you can grow plants?

This was the start of a conversation with my inner teachers, seven groups of consciousness I call my Councils, that has continued for upward of fifty years. They have provided me not just with channeled information but also with an intensive experiential training in exploring consciousness itself. The root of this training focused on helping me understand that we are multidimensional beings who span a spectrum from spirit to mind to body — and beyond. Healing ourselves involves being able to step in and actively co-create the body-mind in alignment with the spirit. Among the Councils' members were healers and teachers from many traditions, including shamanic and earth-based ones. Thus, much of the guidance was in the form of activities, explorations, and experiences — very down-to-earth.

After learning about consciousness and energy medicine through intense training with my inner teachers, through practice as an energy healer and channel with more than ten thousand clients and students, and, since 2007, through study with energy medicine pioneer Donna Eden, I have come to see energy dialogue via the body not only as key to healing my own *dis-ease* and ailments but also as a doorway through which each of us can learn how to create personal, social, and planetary well-being.

In this book, I am showing you how to find this doorway within yourself and inviting you, in your own ways, to step through it.

Energy medicine is the practice of communicating with yourself using the language of energy. You are made of energy; your body communicates with itself using energy; and your actions and choices are fueled by energies as well. You are essentially a matrix of swirling, intertwining subtle forces, not the solid "thing" your mind perceives.

The guidance I get when I tune in to my body taps into this energetic exchange. What I receive is not always in words, and it isn't usually philosophical beliefs or platitudes. It arises in pictures and direct knowing, feelings and sensations, nudges or clear understandings. It comes to me in the language my body speaks: energy. And I try to respond in kind, communicating not just with thought or words but energetically, with movement, gesture, image, sound, smell, sensation, activity, and more.

When you can tap into all that communication through energetic exchange and partner with your own subtle energies, you will find yourself able to heal most anything. Beyond that, you will discover your own individual ways to be well and flourish.

This seems like a big promise. But it is really just common sense:

- If you can communicate with yourself and within yourself, you can activate the amazing internal guidance system built into how we are structured to determine what you need moment by moment.
- You can also make clearer choices about what you do and how you do it.
- When you can communicate this way, your body feels heard and supported and stops shouting at you with symptoms.
- In addition, your stress levels drop, because you are aligned within yourself, from inner truth through outer expression.
- Your body can then use its resources to heal rather than needing them to cope with stress.

- The "instructions" that allocate resources and guide your body to function shift to actively support well-being rather than dis-ease.
- This fuels you to develop your gifts and fulfill your potential.

An unexpected benefit of learning to hear body guidance is that it opens you and provides the instrument for hearing the guidance of your Wiser Self and Councils as well.

Your inner guidance system is not just a right-answer machine, telling you, "Yes, do this" or "No, avoid that." It is also not just a place to seek higher spiritual guidance from your Councils, though that is valuable. It is a form of inner wisdom, built into the instrument that is your body, specific to you as a soul having a human experience. It's a source of ongoing specific and pertinent insight about what is happening within your creation of self and world — what is needed, what is intended, what is viable or unsustainable, and so on. It's there to help you see more clearly, choose more wisely, and experience more fully.

And it is the doorway to everything: healing, fulfilling your soul's potential, peace, radical change.

Why is it important to get to know this guidance system and access this doorway? Increasingly, all of us are being buffeted by shifts in our circumstances, thinking, and the world as we know it. This deeply affects our ability to heal, be well, and evolve our bodies (and social structures) to handle new situations. If I can't tune in to my inner guidance system for truth and clarity about my own soul's choices, I am at the mercy of the swirling winds of change and the theories, competing beliefs, and even slippery "facts" of our present time. Inner guidance acts as a crucial anchor in times of uncertainty.

Radical change is likely to be the theme of our shared reality for some time to come. I think it is ironic that 2020 was the year when crazy worldwide upheaval manifested in the form of a global pandemic, social disruption, collapse of infrastructure, and collision between autocracy and the voice of the people — 2020, which for eyes means perfect vision!

Around 2010, one vision my inner teachers offered was that we were entering a new era that would be ushered in by at least thirty years of radical change. The word *radical* derives from the Late Latin word *radicalis*: "forming the root, inherent." And so radical change is not so much about altering the outer conditions or arguing over new policies and rules as it is about experiencing a transformation in our hearts and minds, in our habits and ways of communicating.

From my perspective, that is great news. You can transform the outer world by refocusing your attention on the core. As my Councils put it, "The task is to find the true shift that brings you home when homeless, into safety when threatened, into allegiance when split, into connection with the inner sparks that will fuel this journey."

And they added: "As you learn to do this, you bring others along."

I have come to see this new era as the rise of *empowered yin*. After some ten thousand years of extreme yang — outward-focused growth, evolution, and actions — the tide is turning to pull us inward again, gently leading us to get to know our roots, our receptive and creative side, our ability to gestate new life in the womb of inner awareness.

It is something like a new tooth erupting: we are going to love it when it arrives, but in the meantime, the gums are inflamed, and it is painful to chew.

I grew up in the feminist 1970s, marching to transform the world. We proclaimed, "The personal is political." We pushed as hard as we could for justice. Some things changed, but a lot didn't. The systems that create inequity continued their inevitable advance toward this moment, when they are finally collapsing under their own weight — unsustainable, unaffordable, and unlivable.

Now, the world is changing us. I like to think mother nature let us have our freedom to run amok, to live in disharmony with her and with our creature nature, until this moment. Today, she is inviting us, event by event, to wake up to what we have been doing to our bodies, minds, and spirits. We are being shown how life as we have been living it has affected our physical, mental, spiritual, and societal health and the health of the planet.

What we took for granted, what we considered order, what we thought about ourselves and other people are all coming into question. We are being unmasked, even those of us who felt awakened and evolved. And within that process, mother nature is giving us the opportunity to evolve further and come home to wiser ways of being. I'm not blaming mother nature here for the collapse of societies as we've known them — I am giving her credit!

∽ Play with It! ∽

Put your hands out in front of you, like an old-fashioned balance scale. On one hand put "going back to the way things were." On the other hand put "moving forward to a new configuration." Let your hands shift up and down with the weight of each choice and see which weighs more for you right now.

If your hands showed you "going back to the way things were," get back in bed or find somewhere to be by yourself. Hunker down and try the following sequence:

- Pet yourself like a dog or cat. Start at your temples, one hand on each side of your head. Stroke up around your ear and down behind it, bringing your hands down to squeeze your shoulders. Then return to stroking again, to calm the freaked-out being that wants to scurry back to what felt like security. Good dog! Good kitty! (For a fuller explanation of this exercise, see "Pet the Doggy / Pet the Kitty," pages 101–2.)
- Trace hearts over your anatomical heart to walk back any emotional reactivity you are experiencing.
- Connect in with yourself in very physical ways, intuitively placing your hands wherever they want to be on your body. Use your healing hands to speak fluently to your creature self, consoling and bringing you home.

When you feel ready, keep reading.

If your hands showed you "moving forward to a new configuration," take a moment to think about where your body wants to sit, lie, stand, or move:

- Do you want to be in a certain room, outside in nature, next to a loved one?
- Do you need a certain color around you, to breathe in a certain scent?
- Do you need a particular song playing to accompany you?

Ask what this self needs now and then supply it, even if what you need seems dumb or can only be supplied symbolically. You might use an object from around the house; a talisman; a representative from nature, such as a stone, a flame, a glass of water, a growing plant, or something metal; a gesture, movement, or shift in position; a change in lighting or visuals to look at.

When you feel ready, keep reading.

☖ • ☗

If you want to be more resilient as mother nature throws us curveballs, as we are pushed to grow by fluctuating circumstances, as we wake up to larger realities, then you will benefit from working with the energetics of change. It is time to stop being caught in the vortex of illness, wounding, and brokenness that are often the primary focus of our healing professions. Instead, we each can benefit by shifting our emphasis to proactively building our well-being.

Change is not just a reorientation in ideas, outer details, or the plot of your life. It is a revamping of how you use energy, how you deploy yourself and employ yourself, moment by moment. And it requires you to gain skill in communicating with your body, mind, and spirit using their own language. The good news is that your body, mind, and spirit already speak energy, and your conscious mind can learn to build fluency from that inborn knowledge.

This book will help you use the language of energy to navigate radical change: from chaos to clarity, from being ill to wellness, from watching things fall apart to finding your unique tools to reconfigure the world you want to live in.

HOW TO USE THIS BOOK

Throughout this book you can augment your baseline understandings of the language of energy to gain fluency through:

- Explorations (Play with It!) of how energy works to initiate change
- Stories that awaken you to your own beliefs and experiences
- Energy exercises to help you rebalance and embody change
- Energy protocols that allow you to work on energies in a more complex way
- Guided Visits that teach you how to explore the energy streams that fuel you
- Energy medicine tools to connect you into your instrument and show you how to work with the dynamics of well-being
- Lifestyle medicine that shows you how to bring energy shifts into your everyday moments

Although this book is chock-full of activities, it is designed so you can read it straight through, picking up insights and perspectives from both the narrative and the activities without needing to stop and try each one. On the other hand, the activities are there for a reason, so you can also use the book as a kind of self-exploration guide to initiate you into the mysteries of your inner byways.

There is an inner logic to the order of the chapters (personally, I always read books in order). However, you can use the book as reference too, dipping into the topic that calls to you now or opening it at random to see what the Universe wants to bring to your attention.

The energy medicine exercises and explorations give you specific instructions on how to do them, but most are intended to act like yogurt starter, helping you to create your own personalized energy medicine. The Guided Visits will take you through the warp and weft of your *web of meaning* — the core energies that feed you. They are presented in a form that makes them as readable as possible, but if you want to experience them as narrated visits, so you can shut your eyes and just follow along, you can download MP3 recordings of each one at ellenmeredith.com/visits, password: YBSW.

If you try to read this book as a traditional how-to or instruction manual, you may get frustrated. It is meant to unfold more the way a novel does: with stories and journeys through material that might require you to suspend your expectations until you can experience where it is taking you. The stories are not just case studies illustrating points; they are meant to ring a bell and put you in touch with your own experiences. If you can, try to read this book with both your intuitive and logical brains and let the concepts and language unpack in your mind and activate your own inner knowing.

Chapter One

From the Inside Out

In the early days of spellchecker (before autocorrect), every time I typed my name, Ellen, the computer would query: "Alien?" I'd laugh and ask, "How did you know?"

Growing up in Michigan, I felt like an alien stranded on a strange planet much of the time. I was always laughing at the weirdness of everyday things that we took for granted. I'd sit in school and wonder, *How come there are twenty-five people in this room, all with something to say, and the teacher keeps shushing us and talking on and on?* I'd wonder, *How did someone decide we should talk about Vikings, or Columbus, or the state bird today?*

At home, I'd look at the objects in our house and wonder how they came to be invented. Why did our refrigerator resemble an upright coffin? Why wasn't it round or some other shape? I'd listen to my older sisters and brother bickering about their belongings, and to my parents refereeing, and suddenly I'd see the scene from the outside, a strange ritual whose purpose I didn't understand. I'd wonder what would happen if we all just stopped a minute to decide what we'd really like to discuss. I didn't know what that might be, but I yearned for it.

The rules, patterns, and reality of everyday life felt random to me, sometimes entertaining, but mostly just a strange picture of being human pasted onto something that might be much more vital if we could just get to it.

At times, of course, I was just in the thick of the drama, living it for what it was. But at the edges of my days, I'd ask myself, *Who wrote this play I'm in?*

Some years later, when I started my channeling practice, I was taken aback by how many of my clients wanted to know if they were aliens. Their sense of displacement and disorientation, of *otherwhere*, was so strong that they wanted to find out from their guides if they were in fact from another planet or galaxy or universe. I wasn't sure I even believed in planetary aliens, though as someone speaking for disembodied consciousness, I couldn't rule them out. But I came to respect that feeling of otherwhere as an important opening.

In retrospect, I think that suspicion of being alien was in fact the first stirring of awakening to the ways we co-create the world rather than being born into a fixed universe. My inner guidance system — our inner guidance systems — were readying us for the big shift in consciousness we are now collectively experiencing. It was preparation for many of us to question why we organize our shared reality the way we do and to recognize that we don't fit in because the outer worlds and shared cultures we inhabit are not really set up in ways that will accommodate each of us, with our spectacular gifts and potentials. We are not meant to fit into the world; it is meant to be an expression of us.

If you were born before the year 2000, you most likely experienced the old reality, which I have come to think of as the *outside-in culture*. It was the yang era: reality was created externally through shared beliefs, social patterns, actions, and fixed structures. I am glad I got to experience it so thoroughly, though it means that, like many on the planet during this bridge time, I've had to rethink my notions of reality and truth.

I am also glad to be able to witness and participate in the shift to creating *inside-out culture*: the era of empowered yin, when we are being asked to transcend socially assigned truths and realities, black-and-white either/or thinking, and learn to navigate via an inner compass instead. We are being invited to embrace what I call *both/and thinking*— the recognition that inner truth can generate many diverse outer realities.

As we usher in the new, more yin ways of being and thinking, the goal isn't just to jettison yang thinking. Instead, we transform it, repurposing what is useful about it while shifting how we respond to it. And we bring in the inner compass, the inner knowing and guidance system built into our bodies, to evaluate what needs to be transformed or repurposed.

What does it mean to transform outside-in thinking and live from the inside out?

OUTSIDE-IN THINKING VERSUS INSIDE-OUT THINKING

With outside-in thinking, we are taught to turn to experts to tell us what we need and what is correct.

Outside-in expertise emphasizes knowledge, information, facts. This requires us to believe that generic expertise and objective facts can readily be applied to our individual situations. Sometimes these generic truths do in fact apply to us. But more often they are an uncomfortable garment.

With inside-out thinking, I have an inner compass, an attunement to my inner guidance system, that allows me to know which expertise is relevant to my particular circumstances now.

Inside-out expertise is characterized by asking good questions, having flexibility, knowing how to frame an endeavor. Also, when I'm operating within the inside-out paradigm, I make the time to develop my own expertise, taking others' input into account but recognizing I need a perspective that is tailored to my particular spirit, mind, and body.

Daria stands out in my mind as someone who desperately needed to use inside-out thinking and access her inner guidance system. She was an old friend I hadn't seen for at least ten years who showed up to visit my partner and me in Switzerland. We picked her up at the airport and helped her drag three huge, heavy suitcases to the car.

I was surprised by how Daria looked. She was extremely well-groomed and chic but had large, swollen yellow bags under her eyes and a gauntness I hadn't remembered. Chalking it up to jetlag, we suggested she get to bed early and invited her to join us for an outing the next day.

Daria emerged better rested the next morning but still with the gaunt look and swollen bags under her eyes. After breakfast, we asked, "Ready to go?" and she said, "I just need about forty-five minutes to take my vitamins." This mystified us until she fetched a stack of seven fishing-tackle boxes from her room. She set them up on the table with three large glasses of water and opened the first: it had about forty compartments filled with vitamins. We watched in horror as she proceeded to swallow pills from each of those compartments, working her way through all seven tackle boxes, swallowing upward of three hundred pills!

Then, without a word, she bundled the boxes back into her room and proclaimed herself ready to go.

At that time, I was trying to learn not to give unsolicited advice, so I kept my mouth shut. However, a few hours later, when she was asking about my healing work, she said, "Do you know why I have these yellow bags under my eyes?"

The words "vitamin poisoning" leapt unbidden from my lips. I tried to make it sound less judgmental: "It may be that your liver can't handle so many vitamins at the same time. Did some practitioner recommend you take all of those?"

"Oh, yes," she said, "my naturopath."

"All at once?"

She looked surprised that I would ask that. "No, over the years."

I suggested mildly that the naturopath probably didn't intend the suggestions to be additive and that she should perhaps take only the five most relevant ones and hold off on the rest until her next appointment.

Daria was not stupid. She had a PhD in psychology. But no one ever taught Daria how to ask her body which supports it needed when, so she bought into the notion that experts could tell her how to be healthy. She applied the notion of "good nutrients" indiscriminately, thinking in distinctly yang-culture logic that if some was good, more would be better.

She was not alone. "Wellness" is a $4.5 trillion business, much of it focused on selling products and devices purported to make you well. It largely pushes health inputs as the path to well-being. And she believed that since her naturopath, an expert, had told her to take the supplements, they were good for her. Even when her body screamed, "Stop!," she couldn't hear it, because she was schooled to follow the advice of outside experts (inaccurately, it turns out) and didn't know how to hear the inner expertise and feedback of her body.

In outside-in thinking, we are trained to seek gratification through external recognition, praise, or fame that validates our membership in society.

In the yang world, our experiences and perceptions must be recognized by others in order to be considered real. We are more valued if we participate in so-called high-status activities. But in that system, value is usually measured in abstract ways: via money, possessions, size, or the ability to sway groupthink.

With inside-out thinking, I am gratified by my own lived experience, whether or not it is meaningful to others.

If I'm living from the inside out, I celebrate my connections with others, shared successes, and individual accomplishments on their own terms and only secondarily in terms of their value to others. I value the essence of what I have offered to the world, and my experience of offering it, over its demonstrated impact on others.

Maya was an MD who came from a long line of doctors. She was happy to join the family tradition, never really questioning it, and she basked in the praise she got from family and mentors as she aced her training and rose rapidly in her profession. At the age of thirty, she was earning great money, respected by her peers, and thinking about starting a family.

But after a two-week bout with a virus, her body began to act up in mysterious ways. She had traveling aches and pains and days when her energy was so crashed out that she couldn't get out of bed. She went for extensive blood work, but nothing out of the ordinary showed up. Along with her doctors, she assumed the symptoms would just fade with time. But they didn't; they worsened, until she was in pain most of the day and none of the medications she tried helped. She finally ended up taking a leave from and then quitting her medical practice.

She suffered in that twilight breakdown for several years, eventually finding the will to try an alternative approach, seeking help with energy medicine. What pushed her out of her outside-in comfort zone was realizing she could miss out on having children if she didn't do something different. Maya spent much of her first session with me apologizing for being there, because it was such a leap for her to break free from her family programming, which valued the allopathic model as the only valid approach.

Maya could describe in detailed physiological terms how her body behaved, as if it were something she was observing. But she couldn't tune in and feel much beyond the pain. She needed to learn to connect into her body; ask it what it needed, moment by moment; and understand the answers it gave her. And she needed to mourn the loss of her official identity as a successful doctor and allow herself, first, to just not know who she was and, eventually, to discover who she wanted to be from the inside out. This process, of rebuilding her attunement and then her identity from the ground up, healed her body.

This inside-out approach helped Maya reinvent herself and allowed her to break free from the blanket belief that being a doctor gave her meaning in order to find out what, if anything, *within* medicine gave her meaning. Too often in our culture, we ask children, "What do you want to be when you grow up?" (an outside-in way of thinking about goal setting) instead of asking, "What makes your heart sing?" (an inside-out approach to cultivating meaning). When Maya made the shift to explore what made her heart sing in specific moments, her body stopped screaming at her, she opened to a larger world of possibilities, and she healed.

Outside-in perspective dissects the workings of the body-mind down to the granular level and tries to determine the correct inputs to engineer health, wealth, and well-being.

We are encouraged to see the body as an object, maybe a complex machine, and to find the perfect inputs of nutrition, exercise, sleep, and activity that allow our machines to really hum.

Similarly, in the outside-in world we are taught that our mind and spirit need to be tamed and cultivated. We are offered methods to reprogram our minds to hold only positive beliefs about how we can be a successful person, and we are encouraged to pursue spiritual practice almost as a commodity, as a means to enhance our ability to excel in the world.

Inside-out thinking invites me to awaken to and interact with the dynamics of my inner workings, to the moving dance of well-being, health, and abundance, rather than trying to find the correct inputs.

Inside-out thinking allows me to appreciate imperfections, enjoy messiness, embrace mistakes, and try various possibilities to see how they affect me rather than looking for the scientifically "correct" answer. I learn to define health, not in terms of inputs and outcomes, but in terms of how well I can learn from and collaborate with my body, mind, and spirit. If I can focus on the whole spectrum of existence, from soul to mind to body to world and the messy exchanges that happen between these dimensions, this supports my evolution as an embodied soul.

∽ Play with It! ∾

Print out or draw an outline of a person, representing you. Then, using colored pencils or pens, create a doodle map of your inner reality at the moment. As you draw, use shapes and colors and whatever arises in your mind or emerges from your hand to let your subconscious symbolically depict what is in your internal world and how it is moving today. Turn off your controlling brain and let instinct just guide your choice of colors and shapes, fill and emptiness.

Then take a look at what your inner instincts are showing you. What is the feeling tone of the picture (calm, agitated, busy, quiet, active, receptive, et cetera)? If you've drawn shapes, are they closed or open, moving or still? Do they speak to you symbolically? Do the colors or shapes remain contained within the outline you started with, or do they extend beyond its borders?

This is a wonderful exploration to do daily as a way to tune in to yourself, capture something about your mood or energies, and track that learning over time. It helps you to connect with your inner dynamics (an inside-out approach) rather than seeking to dissect and correct yourself (the outside-in norm).

∽ • ∾

In outside-in thinking, we are taught to measure illness by what the thermometer, blood pressure cuff, or blood tests tell us, because we believe objective measures of reality are the only accurate way to know what is going on with our bodies.

In extreme outside-in thinking, we don't believe our body when it tries to signal problems unless some doctor "proves" it is real, using scientific measures.

Inside-out thinking pulls me inward to assess and get a more holistic understanding about what's needed and what's off-balance.

I listen to my own experience, sometimes recognizing it is a distorted guide, to find my way home to my inner sense of truth. Although not everything I experience is objectively true, I can use the subjective as a springboard to recognize what my body, mind, and spirit are trying to communicate. I use outer measures to confirm or expand the conversation I am having as I co-create my body, mind, and spirit.

Bee felt there was something going on with her heart. It felt off to her. She'd tune in to the beating and feel something was blocking the motion. She was worried enough that she went to her doctor and had a whole workup, but nothing showed up on any of the scans or tests. She was told her heart was fine.

But it didn't feel fine, and she developed a headache that wouldn't lift. It felt as if her blood was straining to circulate in her system. She also started to suffer from what she called "brownouts." She would just catch herself waking up from a brown study, with no memory of what had happened for the past ten minutes or so.

All of this sense of "offness" weighed on her. She *knew* her body was trying to tell her something, so she went back to her doctor, received another level of tests, and was again told there was nothing wrong with her.

But her body, mind, and emotions kept telling her something was very wrong. So she decided to travel into her heart with her awareness and ask it what was going on.

She watched her breathing for several minutes, then followed the inhale inside, until she felt like she was sitting inside her heart itself. She asked, "What's going on?" She expected to see something like a blocked artery. Instead, in the corner of her heart, she saw her twenty-one-year-old son, Jake, bent over double in pain. Her sense was that it was not an emotional woe but something physical. She asked, "Will you let me help you?" He nodded, and she gave him a hug and returned to her normal consciousness.

She called Jake immediately. Although usually when she asked him how he was, he just blew her off, this time he said, "I've had an ache in my gut coming and going for the last several months, no big deal, but today I can barely stand up straight. And my head hurts." Jake was not the type of kid to go for help, but Bee said, "I'm coming to get you, and we are going to get this checked." He didn't even make a token objection.

This time, Western medicine was helpful. Jake's medical workup showed he had an infection in his intestine that had moved into his appendix, which was in danger of bursting. He was able to have an endoscopic surgery that evening. By the next morning, Jake was on his way to recovery — and Bee's symptoms had cleared.

Bee's doctor had no objective way of knowing that her symptoms were not emanating from her own body but were in fact a message from her body to grab the attention of her conscious mind. Like those dogs that smell cancer, Bee's body was able to pick up a disease process in her son's body, and because she had learned some tools of inside-out thinking, she was able to travel inside to understand the signals. In the yang perception, we appear separate and distinct. But in yin understanding, we are all inter-connected and can use the web of connections to support one another.

Outside-in thinking has taught us to ask, when sick or upset, "What is wrong, and how do I fix it?"

We want a diagnosis. We want a pill or treatment and preferably a quick fix. We focus in on the problem area, where the pain lives, and look for invaders or broken equipment. We go to specialists who attend only to the specific area, and we don't expect them to think holistically.

Inside-out thinking teaches me to use cultivation of plants as a model, to ask, "What do I need to plant in my garden in order to thrive, and how can I cultivate it?"

In this mode, I see things going wrong as a result of what I've planted or as a breakdown in how I am tending to my own cultivation of mind, body, and spirit. I look for ways to shift how I am using and supporting the garden to take the pressure off the problem areas and allow them to heal. I work with the patterns of nature and let the situation unfold in its season.

Our challenges are rarely events of the moment. They are problems that develop over time, in stages or phases. They are usually problematic in context: they keep us from living the life we want to live, from enjoying our experience, from fulfilling our visions or hopes.

Too often we want to flatten them down to a single formulation: What's wrong, and what can I do to fix it? This assumes that the "it" has a single cause and single effect, which is rarely true.

Instead, it is helpful to ask your body for guidance: "What season is it? What phase am I in with my problem or situation or challenge?"

∞ Play with It! ∞

Explore treating your challenge like a planting. I was bemoaning something that had gone wrong in my digestion one day. My Councils said, "If you want cauliflower in your garden, you need to plant cauliflower in the spring." What they meant was that I needed to pay attention to caring for my digestion (and the garden it grows in) at all stages — and not just when something went wrong with it!

I asked my body what season I was in with my digestion. I got the answer: winter. So I realized I needed to let my digestive system rest, maybe mend my tools by thinking differently about food or eating. I needed to envision a different relationship with digestion. I could apply everything I knew about winter to respond appropriately to my digestive woes. Following the wheel of the seasons showed me how to heal this rather complicated issue over time.

Try it yourself. Select a situation you are concerned about: an illness, a problem in your relationship, a challenge at work.

Keeping that situation in mind, ask your inner guidance, "What season is it?" Using your arm as a gauge can help your mind "hear" what your inner guidance has to say. Picture a clock in front of you. Imagine your arm is the arm of that clock and, holding it straight, point it downward to six o'clock, the fallow or winter season.

Very slowly begin to bring your extended arm (you can use either arm) sweeping upward in a clockwise circle, circling up on the left and down on the right. Pay close attention to where your arm moves comfortably and where it wants to stop.

Don't think about where it "should" stop. Just let your body show you where it wants to stop and notice anything you can about how your arm moves along the way. Where are the sticky points? The places where your arm moves smoothly? Where did it finally land?

Your arm should stop, or lose energy, in the position that corresponds to what season you are in with your situation or challenge:

- Six on the clock, arm pointing downward, is winter.
- Nine on the clock, arm pointing left, is spring.
- Twelve on the clock, arm pointing upward, is summer.
- Three on the clock, arm pointing to the right, is fall.

Positions in between indicate times in seasonal transition.

Then, spend some time thinking about your situation or challenge in relation to the position in the wheel of the seasons your body showed you. Let yourself reflect on how the symbolic and energetic truth of each season (and positions in between) speak to your present experience. What can it tell you about what you need and how to best support yourself right now? Bring your own experiences with plant processes of growth to this activity.

You can use the following guide to assess what your body has communicated. The positions on the circle (as if you are looking at the clock in front of you) are shown in figure 1.1.

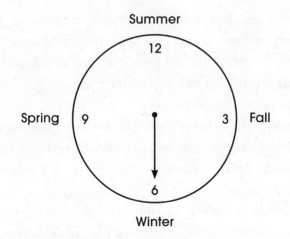

Figure 1.1. The circle of the seasons

Seasonal Energies

Winter is the fallow period, when apparently nothing grows. It is a time of rest, waiting, staying inside, repairing tools. The whole plant consolidates its resources at this time, though often winter brings plenty of moisture to feed the root system. Nutrients from the fallen, rotting leaves seep down to feed the soil. It is often a time when we envision and plan the garden we want to plant in the spring. And in late winter, we sometimes sprout seedlings indoors, in anticipation of being able to move them to the garden in late spring.

Spring is a time of much activity: preparing the ground, spreading mulch, aerating the soil, and then in late spring planting seeds or seedlings. It is a time when the sun gets stronger and brighter. In early spring, we are generally more focused on the field or ground than on the individual plants, which are not yet visible or significant. They are unfurling from the seed, setting roots, anchoring at this time. We are weeding, watering, keeping them protected from insects as they grow. But then, as spring proceeds, plants push outward, expand, produce pollen, and fill in.

Summer is when the crops grow most vigorously, flourishing and showing their personalities. Depending on the plants, some put out fruits, flowers, or nuts, ripening into forms that can nourish us. Summer is often when we are most clearly interdependent with the garden, cultivating food to eat and supporting plants as they produce successive crops. It is also a time when the plants need protection from overly strong sun and from insects, critters, and others who are interdependent with the same garden.

Fall is when we bring the final harvests in, and the growth of the past few seasons falls off to decay and enrich the soil. It is when plants often die back or get cut back. The days shorten, and weather grows cooler. It is often a time to plow things under, let go, celebrate what has been, and face the death of this growing cycle. It is a time when people throw harvest festivals to thank mother nature for her bounties.

Note: you can adjust these descriptions to match the seasons as you know them.

∞ • ∞

With outside-in thinking we are taught to build our life as an edifice and to accumulate wealth to sustain that edifice. We believe that structures and wealth give us security.

In that context, change is often a nuisance rather than a renewal, especially personal change. We put paid work at the center of our identity and too often evaluate experience in terms of how it will affect our résumés. We value "productive" activities that garner wealth, such as being an entrepreneur, more than we value play or sustaining activities, such as caregiving, nurturing, support. We are taught from an early age to compete with others and to celebrate winners, accepting the notion that there will be winners and losers.

With inside-out thinking, I recognize that change is constant. I look for vehicles I can use to get where I need to go, instead of trying to construct permanent structures and stockpiling resources to keep those structures going.

I also value paths that are not necessarily linear — that take me to places I didn't expect to go, places where I can learn, evolve, and deepen my experience of being an embodied soul.

Florence had five marriages end and moved around a lot. She always beat herself up for not being able to sustain a lasting relationship. She told herself she was bad with love. In moments of clarity, though, she could see why she had chosen each man and did admit to having learned a lot in the process. She still yearned for a marriage like her older sister Cindy's.

Cindy married her high school sweetheart, stayed in their hometown, and raised two kids. From Florence's perspective, Cindy had done everything right and had a secure, meaningful life. And she, Florence, had somehow messed up. She equated the impermanence of her moves and marriages with failure.

Then Cindy was diagnosed with stage 3 breast cancer. At first, Florence felt Cindy was doing that perfectly as well. She'd signed on for everything her doctors recommended: surgery, chemo, radiation. But in one phone call, when Florence told Cindy how much she admired her strength, Cindy broke down sobbing and couldn't stop. Florence told her, "I'll be on a plane tomorrow."

The reality Florence discovered when she arrived to take care of Cindy through her treatment process was that the perfect marriage was a perfect facade. It is true, Cindy and her husband had some meaningful history, but as she confessed, the relationship had degenerated to a "ship without much relating." Her husband shut down in the face of her illness and was spending long hours at his office, implying falsely that without these efforts the family would founder financially. They had plenty of money, but the truth was, they had never found their rhythm as a couple once the kids no longer needed them to be a cohesive family.

Florence insisted on bringing Cindy to me for energy medicine sessions as a complement to her conventional medicine approaches. With Cindy's permission, she sat in on the sessions to learn what she could do to help. What she discovered was that in the years she had been forced to deal with loss and change and failure of love, her sister had clung to a reality that was not sustaining her in the least. And Cindy, who had also bought into the myth of her happy life and Florence's chaotic one, had to unlearn a form of passivity that Florence could never have afforded, given her life challenges.

Florence got to see firsthand that security was not conferred by outer circumstances but was a state of mind. Together, the sisters made a pact to change what they needed to change, but also to put their dreams more at the center of their lives.

Florence decided to move to Oregon, which she thought would suit her personality better than the "nowhere" town she had landed in after her most recent marriage. And she joined a cohousing community, realizing that whether or not she had a love interest, she could build a web of relationships that might give her a sense of belonging.

Cindy went into remission from the cancer and with Florence's help was able to break through the denial that was holding her life in stasis. She decided to stay in the marriage for the time being, as a baseline, while she actively sampled other experiences that might help her figure out what would make her heart sing.

�)•(☺

What do you need in order to transform your life from the outside-in yang beliefs that still dominate our shared culture to yin-supportive practices? There is no fixed formula for healing and living from the inside out . . . beyond learning to do it.

But the following chapters do offer energy tools and practices that can support you in this transformation. They include:

- Waking up to the ways that prioritizing yang values, outer forms, and impacts keep you from healing, being well, and thriving
- Learning to work more skillfully with your own individual guidance system to let your body show you the way to meet the rising pull toward inside-out living
- Learning to show up for yourself and actively co-create the moments and frameworks that best express your spirit
- Learning to speak energy more fluently in dialogue with the

energies of your body, mind, and spirit and to deepen from
dialogue to conversation

- Learning to work with the syntax of the language of energy —
the patterns by which you create a self and participate in the
shared web of connections
- Learning to work with the key dynamics of creating a self —
gatekeeping, grounding and anchoring, coherence, flow,
exchange between self and world, and radiance — as you navigate today's rising tide of ongoing and radical change

∽ Chapter Two ∾

Rename, Reframe, and Reclaim

Many years ago, Anne went traveling in Asia to visit sites sacred to Quan Yin, a feminine form of the Buddha. After she got home she developed a red, angry infection down in her private area. It itched, then it hurt, then itched and hurt. The whole area was swollen and driving her crazy.

She consulted a tropical medicine specialist, but he couldn't figure out what was wrong. They checked multiple times for parasites and didn't find any; they even tried some broad-spectrum medications to wipe the infection out, but to no avail.

So she consulted a dermatologist and tried different salves. The dermatologist kept saying, "It could be thousands of things. Try this." Nothing worked.

She then went for acupuncture and drank some off-putting herbal concoctions but got no relief. The condition came and went for months and seemed to have a mind of its own.

Anne was a dedicated Buddhist whose trip to Asia had been a pilgrimage to deepen her practice. Whatever benefits she had gained from the trip were rapidly receding as she became more and more preoccupied

27

with how to deal with the inflammation. She was enraged that her life and dedication to her spiritual practice were being derailed by this pain and discomfort.

Finally, she asked herself the question: *What do I know that I could bring to bear on the situation?* Her answer: "I have my Buddhist practice. Instead of trying to get rid of this pain and avoid it, I'm going to befriend it. I'm going to turn toward it."

You know those Chinese puzzles that are straw tubes and when you stick your fingers in both ends, your fingers get stuck? Spoiler alert: the solution is to push inward, and your fingers release. That's essentially what she did with this illness. She pushed inward. She leaned into it.

The first step was that she recognized she had to stop jokingly referring to it as "the plague." She decided to tune in and ask its name. She dropped into meditation, centered on the affected area, and asked, "What should I call you?" She heard: "Blanche."

Anne thought this was hilarious, since *blanche* means "white," and this was a very red, angry thing.

Her second step was to ask, "Blanche, what do you need? How can I serve you?" She added, "I'm not going to try to get rid of you. I'm going to find out what you're here to teach me."

She started interacting with this new friend whenever symptoms showed up. If she was planning to go to a party and the red, angry itch appeared, she'd stop and say, "Oh, B., what do you need? What can I do for you?" Blanche might give her the image of taking a cold sitz bath to cool her down. Anne would say, "OK." She'd take off her party clothes and sit in the bath.

Or she'd be sitting down to eat, and symptoms would flare up and she'd say, "B., what's going on?" She'd tune in, and her attention would be drawn to something on her plate. She knew it meant, "Don't eat that. I don't want that." Anne would put the food away and get something else that Blanche would signal was more to her liking.

Anne got very nuanced at this dialogue because her Buddhist training had taught her to tune in and really notice subtleties. She began to enjoy the challenge of responding appropriately, in ways Blanche could understand.

About three weeks after Anne committed to the dialogue, Blanche was gone, never to return again. Anne was healed because she allowed her body, via this collaboration, to teach her what she needed to know. In the process she deepened her spiritual practice in a very physical way.

WHAT'S IN A NAME?

Anne never got a clear diagnosis of what Blanche would be called in medical terms. It was frustrating not to know what it was. However, in many ways that lack of a diagnosis, of a medical name, freed Anne to show up and find ways to encounter the situation on its own terms.

Whether or not you have an official diagnosis of your illness, or your relationship woe, or your work problem, or your social challenge, think about how having a name for it shapes your understanding, for good and for bad.

When a doctor says you have "cancer," that taps into a whole energy field associated with the word *cancer*. You have associations from people you've known with cancer, some of whom probably died from it or were permanently scarred by the extreme treatments, which adds a layer of fear and alarm to your experience. Seeing your situation as part of the larger phenomenon of "cancer" (irrespective of what kind, since the word is used to describe dozens of different diseases) can set off a whole cascade of biochemical, energetic, emotional, behavioral, and physical reactions in you.

But cancer is not a thing. It is a name for how cells behave in a whole host of situations. Describing cancer as a dynamic rather than a thing, you might say it is a cell or set of cells that are replicating unnaturally or unable to regulate their growth. They are cells with boundary issues.

Zach Bush, MD, an endocrinologist who works holistically with illness, has a lovely definition of a cancer cell: "What is cancer, ultimately? Cancer, it turns out, is a cell that has forgotten it is part of a larger organism." He talks about a cancer cell as a cell that has lost track of its tribe and, in the panic of finding itself alone, reverts to trying to save its "species" and repopulate by replicating more rapidly. It is a cell with communication and membership issues.

This is logical; it makes sense. And much of what happens in our bodies, minds, and shared social dramas has a logic to it, a story line that will give you clues about how to work with it energetically and behaviorally. When you can get past what you think you know about the diagnosis, the named disease, the phenomenon as it has been depicted in the literature, and find a way to dialogue with the situation on its own terms — not as everyone's "cancer," or "cheating husband," or "dysfunctional workplace" — you can often find wise ways, and personally appropriate ways, to show up and respond.

When we flatten our understanding of situations to a single label or name, particularly one that was assigned by other people, we get caught in collective understandings that may or may not apply to us. When we treat a phenomenon as a named thing, we can easily lose track of the particular energy dynamic going on for us — the very dynamic that is our teacher and that will suggest wise action.

Anne's body knew how to heal what was going on for Anne, once she worked with Blanche to give herself what she needed energetically, nutritionally, and in terms of how she used her energies from moment to moment. Her body guidance might have pulled her to seek out antibiotics or other Western medical help as well, as Bee's did when her son was suffering an infection. But in this case, the inflammation was a signal from Anne's *gatekeeper* (her energetic, physical, mental, emotional, and spiritual immune system) that Anne's body needed a different pattern of care. So when she changed that pattern, her body's energies and chemistry shifted and healed.

As I said above, having an official name for your problem can be both good and bad.

If you struggled long and hard to finally get a diagnosis for something that has been plaguing you, this discussion might seem opposite to your experience. I've had thousands of clients express their relief at finally knowing what was going on medically.

But for many, the relief was short-lived when they were told by Western doctors there was no cure or told by complementary practitioners that the only cure was a strictly regimented diet and thousands of dollars' worth of supplements. For some, Western medicine and complementary medicine did offer treatments that addressed the illness. But in most cases, those treatments carried a lot of damage with the cure. And they did not engage the client in learning to truly communicate with their own instrument and participate in creating their own well-being.

The invitation here is not to dump diagnoses or ignore the real help you can get from professionals in understanding (even treating) what is going on for you. Instead, the invitation is to add in a willingness to show up, find a name that does not carry the baggage of everyone else's experience, dialogue with your body on its own terms, and let it show you, in more holistic ways, how to heal and be well.

Ꮗ Play with It! Ꮗ

Focus in on some challenge you're dealing with. It might be an illness or other physical issue, but it might also be a relationship problem, a difficulty at work, or even something in how your mind works or how you behave that you want to get to know as it plays out for you. This challenge might have a socially recognized name (arthritis, constant bickering, micromanaging, ADHD), or it may be a mystery to you still. Remember, we don't have to accept either/or thinking. We can embrace many ways to understand and name the same phenomenon.

1. **Tune in to your body, focusing on the challenge, and ask for a name.** The trick with this is to avoid trying to *assign* a name or trying to find a name that is a *descriptor*. You are listening for an actual name, such as Fred or Dolores, or a word that can serve as a name, such as Jammy or Butt-Thump.

   It is tempting to look for something noble or meaningful. Or to name it the way you'd name a new puppy, by looking for what fits. But since you are asking this situation to teach you, put aside your desire to shape it and let it introduce itself — and possibly surprise you. Sometimes it will make you laugh or will seem random or silly. But often it will feel significant somehow, even if you don't yet understand why.

2. **Ask Butt-Thump to show you one thing she needs right**

now. This dialogue happens most fruitfully if you can use the whole language of energy and don't try to limit it to a verbal exchange. Butt-Thump might give you an image, sensation, or thought; she might draw your attention or make you feel pulled toward something; she might even activate or intensify one of the symptoms. You might hear words or just know directly.

If you are not used to this kind of dialogue, you might not "hear" or perceive anything right away. Just keep asking and staying open to how your body wants to guide you. Often if you get nothing, it is because you are actually asking, "What's wrong?" You want to know the cause or what it needs in order to go away rather than authentically asking how you can bring support to your body right now. Guidance in the present is often quite simple: *rest, sit down, stretch your muscles, let go, breathe.*

Remember, this isn't about asking for right answers. Just ask for insight about what your situation or body needs energetically, materially, and in terms of attention, care, and action in the moment.

3. **Play with your associations.** What does the name mean to you? Often I get a name and later realize it is perfectly symbolic or carries meaningful associations. Butt-Thump might make you realize you feel like you've been kicked in the rear. Dolores might make you realize sadness is an element. Or you might play with the word and think, *Duh — lores,* as in, *Hey, dummy, this is family lore playing out again.* Fred might make you think of Fred Flintstone, an angry, reactive cartoon character. In my mind, I associate Fred with peace, because it is the word for peace in Norwegian. It is not cheating to look up the roots of your new name, to see what it derives from or means linguistically. We often carry these associations in our subconscious, which sends our conscious mind names that are more apropos than we might realize at first.

4. **Stay open and focus on getting to know Butt-Thump, as you**

would get to know a new acquaintance. What does she like or dislike? How does she behave in various circumstances? How do her energies play out, and what are the dynamics of her presence in your life? Illness isn't a discrete consciousness, but it is a fragment of your consciousness you can connect with, get to know, and befriend.

5. **As Fred, Dolores, Jammy, or Butt-Thump communicates, learn to respond appropriately, moment by moment.** This newly named situation doesn't necessarily have all the answers. Their main job is to give you access to specific insight about the dynamics and nature of your challenge and what might be needed. If you get the message to jump off a bridge, you don't just go jump off a bridge! You need to investigate what is being communicated. Is your body expressing despair, a feeling of being trapped in a transition, or maybe even yearning to leap into the void and experience something new?

    Your appropriate response is to recognize the intent within the communication and honor it in some way. So, for example, the appropriate response to despair is to offer hope or connection, not to just jump off the bridge.

    Appropriate response may be physical: eating or avoiding certain foods, massaging or stretching parts of your body, shifting position, dancing, resting. It may be energetic: doing some energy medicine exercises or lifestyle medicine (everyday activities that influence your energy) to help your body shift its balance. It might be emotional: consoling the despairing being, validating the feelings that are arising. It may be behavioral: changing what you do or how you do it. And it may be symbolic: you may need to make an artwork or create a ritual to enact that truth for yourself.

6. **Continue to dialogue with and learn from Butt-Thump, until she moves on or you have integrated her lessons into your larger understanding of what being well means for you.** Example: One day recently, I had a mild migraine. I have a long history with migraines, including a period of

fifteen years of daily ones. So rather than ask myself, "Why am I getting another migraine?" I asked, "Hmm, who just showed up?" I tuned in and heard the name Hortense. I asked Hortense what she needed from me right now. My hands lifted to cover my ears. This made me start yawning uncontrollably. So I shut my eyes and kept yawning, letting it develop into breathing from my diaphragm. I asked if I could do anything else for her. My attention was drawn to my feet, which felt like solid lumps of clay. I took a few moments to work the clay, loosen it, open up the energies of each part of my foot. As I did this, I felt the inflammation in my head receding.

I spent a few minutes wondering who Hortense was. My previous migraine had been named Minerva. I played with "whore-tense," but that didn't fit. Then I realized that I associate the word *hors* with the French, meaning "outside," as in *hors service*: "out of service." And then I remembered that before Hortense showed up, I was noodling through an online newspaper and reading about racist laws and lawmakers. The stress of that *hors tense*, or "outside tension" — tension I didn't need on that particular day at that particular moment — probably triggered the arrival of Hortense as a physical communication.

I decided to avoid reading the news in the midst of my day and focus on it only when it was a conscious choice. Hortense did not return until a few weeks later, when I again slipped into letting the outside news infiltrate my day without consciously choosing it. I needed only a twinge of headache to realize I'd forgotten to maintain that particular self-protection.

Even though I still sometimes use the socially loaded term of *migraine*, experientially I've gotten to understand the energetic dynamics of what makes my head *go out* through the teachings of Hortense, Minerva, Myron, and others. And they have helped me to trust that my body is not just going haywire. There is purpose and communication in what I experience. If I can let this situation show me its dynamics, reveal what is playing out energetically, I can communicate purposefully in response, and my symptoms either dissipate or show me the next step on the path to healing.

☞ • ☜

REFRAME

Try this experiment. Look around you, letting your vision scan in a 180-degree arc. What did you notice? Now, make a circle with your thumb and index finger and look through it, like a spyglass. Scan the same 180-degree arc with your finger spyglass and notice what you see this time.

When I scan my surroundings in a general sweep, I see very little detail. I get impressions of colors and textures, and I notice wall, picture, curtains, mirror, wall hanging, window. Mostly my mind just names what it sees. But when I view the same room in framed moments, I see the image in the picture in more vivid detail, notice a light my earlier sweep missed and how utilitarian its design is, see the expression on my face in the mirror, and appreciate the lovely curve of a railing on the steps outside my window. In short, I get more information.

Framing shapes how we see something. Often framing also influences how well or how clearly we see something. If you frame your relationship as "falling apart," you might miss details you would notice if you were to frame it as "falling apart so it can reformulate" or "reaching the end of a cycle."

Anne, who used her Buddhist practice to befriend her pain, reframed her health woes by moving from seeing them as a plague to seeing them as a teacher and, further, as Blanche, someone she could get to know. Within this new framework, her understanding transcended the plague aspects of the situation and zeroed in on specific dimensions that ultimately gave her more clarity and awareness of what her body was expressing. It gave her a way to move the situation forward and improve it, whereas seeing it as a plague had been funny but led nowhere.

Framing is a core skill for healing, living well, and being able to thrive.

It is the art of structuring how you see something so that you can actually work with it and make a difference.

"My husband dumped me" may communicate your sense of hurt, but it also puts you squarely in the victim seat and flattens what are probably years' worth of difficult moments you'll want to sort out.

"My husband left, and I'm in the process of trying to reclaim myself" tells your body and hurt self that you aren't a throwaway at the mercy of his unskillful exit. It tells others not to project their breakups and the culture of dumping onto what was probably a much more complicated set of interactions than they know.

Framing is not the same as euphemisms, which avoid calling things what they are with words that are impersonal. And it's not the same as spin, which is about packaging a situation to sell it to others (or to oneself).

Instead, framing has to do with accepting your power to influence and shape your own experience, to assign your own meaning. It offers you a way to bring in your wisdom, to create understandings that help you grow, heal, and evolve, rather than digging you deeper into the culture of illness, wounding, and victimization.

Imagine you go to the store and end up waiting in line for over an hour to get through checkout. How you frame the situation during and after determines your lived meaning of your experience *and how it affects your body*.

If you stand in line fuming, bemoaning your fate of getting stuck in a crowd, and complaining to yourself or others about your bad luck, you create stress on your body and probably poison the experience for other people.

If you disappear into your cell phone and noodle around on the internet, you might be less aggravated about shopping or the store, but on the other hand, your nervous system has to reconcile the two competing realities of electronic stimulation and physical inaction. You might come away feeling vaguely dissatisfied and a bit jumped up energetically.

If you frame the time as a chance to stop momentum and just enjoy where you find yourself, you might strike up an interesting conversation with someone you otherwise would not have met. Or you might choose to use the time to people watch, or to try to figure out how the store operates, or to practice standing meditation, noticing your breath and posture and all the sights and sounds of the store as you practice perceiving.

Each of these choices has a distinct impact on your body and psyche.

And when you report on your experience later, you can tell your loved ones you had a miserable morning, an annoying interlude, a productive time-out, a lovely connection with someone you met, a good laugh at the humanity on display, an edifying observation of how things work, or a good practice time.

Each of these influences how the experience gets stored in your energetic wiring and how your gatekeeper (the keeper of your autopilot) instructs your body and mind to react to future similar situations.

Energy Medicine to Calm Reactivity When Stuck Waiting

Try any of these options:

- **Squeeze or pulse each fingertip at the sides of your fingernail twice, then interlace your hands and place them over your heart or gut.** This activates several of your energy meridians, unscrambles your energies, integrates yin and yang, and brings you back in touch with body wisdom.
- **Cross your arms across your chest.** This helps your energies of left and right brain stay integrated and in touch with your heart.
- **Breathe in on a count of three and out on a count of five for at least a minute.** Exhaling longer than you inhaled allows you to release pent-up energies and calms your vagus nerve, which controls your autonomic nervous system.
- **Ask yourself, *What is each person sacrificing to be here?*** Make up a story for each person you see. This activates your compassion and reinforces your connections with other people.
- **If you are stuck in traffic, squeeze the steering wheel in a very slow, pulsing rhythm, four times on each side, while slowing your breathing. Then tap each foot very slowly four times on each side (not on the pedal!) while breathing slowly.** This stops your need to push toward your destination, sets a rhythm to your waiting, and allows you to be more present.

At each moment, you have the opportunity to choose how you focus, what details you notice, how you engage with life, how you react to (or cope with) involuntary responses, and how you interpret your experience. You also have the opportunity to do something to shift your energies. Because of this, framing is a key to healing and well-being. Many of us walk through life scanning our reality, taking life as it comes, but not actively choosing how to frame our moments.

I am not talking about controlling your moments! There is a positive-thinking movement out there that says, "Only allow yourself to have positive thoughts and feelings." One woman I knew, when asked how she was, would always respond, "Awesome." She would say this whether she was feeling great or was in the midst of dealing with tricky and painful situations. It was difficult for people to *really* know her and to support her appropriately. And, of course, her relentless positivity often turned into denial that made her miss the significance of her own experience.

Even when her husband became ill with a terminal diagnosis, she'd say, "I'm awesome, everything's perfect as it is." That was basically a very fuzzy lens to be looking through! She didn't need to say, "Terrible, I'm freaked out and miserable," though that would have been a valid choice. But she could have framed the situation for herself in a way that would have created an opening for others to connect: "My husband is in the hospital, and I'm trying to understand how I can help him and deal with my own fears right now." She could have framed the situation as: "My husband has a diagnosis that has scared us, and we're trying to stay positive and figure out how to support his body through this challenge."

I'm not suggesting we all become mealymouthed and speak in unnatural phrases. Rather, I'm suggesting that we recognize when the frameworks we choose trigger reaction, defeatism, and judgment in ourselves and others, and that we reframe our situations in ways that can yield better responses.

∽ Play with It! ∾

Write a list of what you would describe as your problems. This is just for your own private exploration, so use your normal, everyday way of speaking. For example, I might write, "I need to lose weight. I don't exercise enough. I have allergies. My friend Sally is annoying, and I don't want to see her anymore."

Then consider each item in turn and explore what frame you used, what that tells you, and how you might reframe the statement.

I start with my theme song, losing weight. Of course, this is what society seems to want most women to do, even skinny ones. So I look at the words: *need, lose,* and *weight.* And I think: *What do I actually need? Why would my body choose to LOSE something? And what purpose does the weight serve? Ballast? Insulation? Evidence of my rebellious nature in not wanting to give in to society's values?*

Now I reframe it and say, "I want to USE weight more skillfully."

In the "lose" frame, I must somehow change my diet, and exercise, and probably deprive myself of the ways I've used food that caused stockpiling. It is a conflict when losing equals success and gaining equals failure.

In the "use" frame, I am looking at how to work more skillfully with how I store energy and appreciate how weight serves me, even if I choose to find different ways to serve the same purpose.

Reframing goes beyond wordplay, though, such as substituting *use* for *lose.* I might also express the situation in a whole new way: "I'd like to fully inhabit my body and live in attunement to her rhythms." This, too, would take me on a journey quite different from one focused on trying to lose weight.

Investigate each of the items on your list and think about how you can reframe them in a way that respects your experience and gives you a path forward.

CO • CO

RECLAIM

Your inner guidance system has an amazing and rich capacity; you can explore it your entire life, and there will still be more to discover. With it, you can attune to the energy exchanges of your body in minute detail, learn to hear what is going on and what is needed, perceive the way your mind and body interact, tune in to other channels, such as planet earth, and also receive the guidance of your Wiser Self and inner teachers. And most of us who grew up in outside-in culture barely know how to use it!

Renaming and reframing support you to *reclaim* your ability to go inward, dialogue with your energies, learn from them in terms specific to you, and activate your body, mind, and spirit's wisdom about how to support the best version of yourself.

I have detailed in my earlier book, *The Language Your Body Speaks: Self-Healing with Energy Medicine,* how to "speak energy" in dialogue with your body, mind, and spirit. There are three particular skill sets that will help you to reclaim your inner guidance system: learning to sense subtle energies; learning to locate the issue or who needs to communicate now; and learning to work energetically with what you discover.

Learn to Sense Subtle Energies

Anne was good with *sensing subtle energies,* so she found it fairly easy to tune in and listen to Blanche's signals. Their dialogue was not merely an inner exchange of words, though sometimes words arose. The relationship with Blanche called on all of Anne's senses, because our senses are a major part of our instrument for receiving information and guidance. If this is not your skill set, it can help you to spend time just going inside and observing what arises in you, as Anne did through her Buddhist practice.

It is useful to break this skill into four steps:

1. **Experience and explore sensations.** Tune in to your physical sensations first (what you see, hear, smell, taste, feel) without trying to interpret or categorize what you are perceiving. There is a difference between feeling something cold, then investigating with an open mind the sensations that arise, versus thinking, *That's cold,* then reacting to the moment on the basis of your previous experiences and mental understandings of cold.

2. **Use your whole vocabulary of experience to characterize what you are picking up.** What does this remind you of? Is there a metaphor or simile that comes to mind? For example,

you may feel tingling sensations and think, *This is like a bunch of ants swarming over decaying food.*

3.   **Explore how you can interact with the sensations you are perceiving.** If your perception is "cold," how do you want to respond to it? If your perception is "a bunch of ants swarming over decaying food," what are your choices? Do you want to wrap the food up and dispose of it, redirect the ants back out into nature? If your instinct is just to kill them or get rid of the sensation, ask yourself, *What or whom am I killing? Does the sensation serve a purpose?*

4.   **Unpack the meaning of your subtle energy communications.** What does it mean to you that you discovered cold in your stomach area? What are your associations with ants swarming over decaying food, and why did you perceive that sensation in that particular part of the body?

Here are a few tips about sensing energies:

- *You already sense subtle energies.* They are part of the radar that allows you to navigate in the realms of body, mind, and spirit. So your goal in this pursuit is to train your mind to *recognize* what it is perceiving. To name it and frame it so the insight or information can serve you.

- *It is useful to keep what I call a Book of Shadows.* This is a journal of the sensations and communications you notice, however fleeting. Just as we can sometimes recognize a form by perceiving its shadow, subtle energies sometimes first appear as wisps of perception. By collecting these in writing, you can begin to see patterns or can unpack the meaning over time.

- *Sensing isn't a static activity, because subtle energies are not static.* When you tune in, you can interact with what you find there, noticing how it moves or morphs or reacts when you touch it. You can interview it and experiment with what happens if you respond with color, sound, image, movement, gesture, or touch.

- Sensing subtle energy starts with recognizing, naming, and framing what is going on with the swirling energies you are made of. Then you may need to *unpack the meaning or recognize the symbolic truth of what is being communicated.* Your subtle energies and senses and consciousness all work together to create meaning.
- *Using your everyday senses and extended senses to perceive how your energy is moving, behaving, and communicating is not primarily about being psychic,* though psychic abilities can arise from learning to sense subtle energies. It is about tuning in to the energies you are made of and interacting with them.

Learn to Locate the Issue
or Identify Who Needs to Speak Now

Are you old enough to remember slide projectors? You would insert an image printed on an acetate square into the machine, and a light would shine through it projecting the picture onto a screen. If you noticed a smudge on the image, you might be tempted to go up to the screen and wipe it away. But most often the smudge was on the slide itself, or inside the projector, or in the air, blocking the clear flow of the image to the screen.

Our bodies are like images projected onto this earthly reality. They appear solid, and they *are* solid in earthly terms. But they are also energetic projections. Too often we try to fix a problem with the body in the place where we see the smudge — in the present, on the body — rather than looking at the slide, the projector, or what might be obscuring the light stream.

Energy healing and, for that matter, well-being are rooted in the understanding of our multidimensional nature. One lesson my Councils have offered me repeatedly over the years is to seek out where a situation I wish to understand emanates from. Where does it live? If I want to dialogue with energies, who am I talking with?

They particularly emphasized that we are not one "thing." We aren't a thing at all. Instead, we are dynamic energies that are most easily understood as having three major densities (with other dimensions also influencing us). These three densities they call:

- **Earth Elemental Self:** the creature self that includes the body and all our animal instincts and earth-oriented wisdom
- **Talking Self:** the mental, imagining self that creates the plot and characters and writes the lines in the dramas we co-create
- **Wiser Self:** the source self, guiding and fueling our earth-based/mind-based reality and bringing in gifts of our nature, unique to each of us

The Councils used these names because, as with all renames, they freed me from the outside-in associations I carried with "body," "mind," and "spirit."

Whenever I'd feel sick or work on a client, one of the first questions I'd hear in my head was: *Where's the projector?* In other words, where is the situation we are trying to address emanating from?

I discovered that it was extremely useful to ask that question and then to call up some energetic sniffer dogs, like the ones that seek out contraband at the airport. I'd call up a sniffer dog and say, "Where's this coming from, Bowser?" Then I'd set Bowser loose to range through the Earth Elemental Self, Talking Self, and Wiser Self dimensions (and elsewhere) to show me where the projector was.

⚭ Play with It! ⚭

Choose a specific challenge you want to explore: a sore body part, a feeling you are having, even an event, like a car accident. Call up an energetic sniffer dog and ask, "Where's the projector?" Follow the dog and note where it takes you. There may be more than one projector, co-creating your situation like a spectacular light show. You can ask the sniffer dog to take you to the most recent projector or to the original projector, if you wish.

Then, sink into the area the sniffer dog signals and explore it using all your senses. Ask that projector or slide for a name and dialogue with it.

Ask it to tell you or show you more about itself, what it needs. And then use whatever energy medicine you know (you'll learn more as you progress in this book) to address what is going on, to clear the smudge where it lives.

∽ • ∽

Exercise: One Hundred Gifts of the Body

Sniffer dogs are usually trained to locate contraband, like drugs, or even illness in the body. But I find they are even more useful in locating gifts and resources! My Councils suggested that I try this exercise:

> Each day, for a period of one hundred days, send a sniffer dog into your body (and energy field and larger self) to locate a gift. Spend the day unpacking the gift, seeing its uses and implications to help your evolution. Write down what you find and what you understand about the gift in a special "One Hundred Days of Gifts" journal. These gifts become steps on a path or pieces of a puzzle that might surprise you in its larger implications. At the very least, they will guide you on a journey.

A gift can be almost anything: a word, an image, a thought, a sensation, a gesture, a direct knowing, or a symbol. The location is often significant as well. Here are some recent gifts that my sniffer dog brought me:

- **Location:** heart. **Gift:** Pledge of Allegiance gesture. I pledged allegiance to myself and found my anxiety about a judgmental colleague lifting.
- **Location:** adrenal glands. **Gift:** image of lotus flowers blossoming from each gland. I tuned in to the energies of those lotus flowers and felt my stress levels receding.
- **Location:** every cell of my body. **Gift:** a Beatles song, "All You Need Is Love." Singing it brought a sense of transcendence throughout my body and calmed an allergic reaction.

- **Location:** end points of stomach meridian (see "Embodiment Stream," pages 174–76). **Gift:** a phrase, "Divest, don't digest." I actually spent several days divesting myself of old stories and beliefs and even getting rid of clothes that didn't fit.

Note: I taught this exercise in a recent class, and students discovered that their sniffers were all kinds of animals, not just dogs. For some of them, the type of animal that showed up with a gift added a level of significance and meaning.

☙ • ❧

I am always struck by the fact that most of the so-called healing in our culture does not happen where our dis-ease lives. It does not happen in the contexts where we live, in keeping with the rhythms we live, nor often even in the part of the body the problem actually emanates from. We submit to a surgery to remove the slide or take a medication to filter out parts of the projected image rather than undertaking a cleanse and rebuild of the projector.

And so a problem that shows up as thyroid disease at one point, reappears as adrenal exhaustion, morphs into a cancer, explodes as divorce, and ripples out through all the dimensions of our being is never adequately addressed because we don't look at where it's emanating from or what it's telling us about how our committee of Earth Elemental Self, Talking Self, and Wiser Self are collaborating.

To free ourselves from the linear thinking that our world seems to love, a key skill is to *ask better questions.* Many of my clients didn't perceive the projectors because they couldn't get past asking, "What is wrong?" and "Why am I sick?" These are natural questions, but the information they yield is about wrongness and sickness, not well-being.

When you get to know another person, the goal isn't to label and pigeonhole them. You learn how their mind works, how they look and respond in different situations, how they sound, how they smell, how you feel in reaction to them. And over time you come to recognize their voice, their moods, their personality, their energies, their style. That's what we want to do with the voices within us, with our body's consciousness itself.

So asking better questions is about conversation and exchange, not about interviewing or testing. And it is about learning to recognize the multidimensionality of responses you receive, especially when they are nonverbal. It is about asking questions that generate lots of potential ("Give me insight into…," "Tell me more about…") rather than questions that winnow everything down to a true/false, yes/no binary.

If you have learned energy testing (see appendix A) as a way to dialogue with your emotions or body, consider whether the binary of yes/no is an adequate vocabulary to truly enlighten you about how your energies unfold. Energy testing can be useful to validate certain perceptions you might have, but it is not a substitute for actual energy conversation.

Learn to Work Energetically with What You Discover

I see my body as a doorway to the infinite, to all the places my mind and spirit can inhabit. And as such, I believe it is a rich place to send the sniffer dogs. My Councils did not just show up in my head to chat or ask me to take dictation. They often introduced a concept like "rename" and then used my life as a workshop to help me unpack its meaning and experience its impacts. Or they took me traveling inside my body or out into other dimensions to get to know energies where they lived.

Once your sniffer dogs show you where the projector is, what can you do with this knowledge? The possibilities are endless, but below is an exercise that you can use as a starting point. Remember my client Bee, whose body was giving her signals about an infection in her son Jake's intestine? Bee had learned this technique in one of my courses and used it to figure out what was going on with her heart. Try this exercise for yourself. You can read the instructions into a tape recorder or download an MP3 recording from ellenmeredith.com/visits, password: YBSW.

Guided Visit: Cradle and Clear an Organ Space

Hold your hands cupped in front of you and imagine you are holding something or someone you treasure: one of your children as a baby, your favorite pet, a beloved crystal. Feel your love for this treasure accumulate in your hands, until you are holding a ball of love.

Take your two love-infused hands and place them over the organ you wish to use as an entry point — for example, over your stomach. Let the love in your hands pour into that organ as you cradle it, the way you cradled your beloved object.

When you feel that the love energy has transferred out of your hands, sink your attention down into the organ, traveling into it the way you would into an inner chamber. For example, if you go down into the stomach organ, take a moment to just tune in to whatever you notice, using any or all of your senses.

For some people, it might be something about the space itself: Maybe the walls seem too tight, the place is dark, or you hear a drip of something leaking. Or maybe the space is wide open, not a chamber at all, but something outdoors.

Don't worry about making the space conform to any expectations. Your job is simply to work with what you find there.

Ask the space for a name. Then ask it what is needed: "Are the walls breached and needing repair?" "Is the energy blocked and needing to be cleared?" "Are there areas where movement is too rapid or too sluggish and need to be adjusted?"

You do not need to see clearly, if that is not your forte. Just notice what you notice. And if you don't perceive anything, use your mind to imagine what might be needed there. Ask the area, "What might be of service to you?"

You can also ask the organ what it needs from you today. Pay attention to whatever enters your mind.

Is it too light or too dark? Is it too hot or too cold? Is it moist enough or too dry? You are not necessarily trying to do a literal repair job on the tissue and vessels (though that is an option). Instead, you are working symbolically with whatever presents itself, using your intention and any tools or materials you would like to request from the Universal Supply Center.

Ask for help or helpers if you need them. Ask for information of the space itself. Don't discard anything that arises, even if you don't understand it. Just use your intuition to address it as best you can.

After you have reached a sense of completion, take a moment to infuse the whole area with something that feels healing to it. Let your intuition guide you on this — it could be something logical, like a color that feels healing; or a nurturing sound; or a soothing gel. But it could also be something that seems a bit strange, like toxin-free antifreeze. As long as it feels emotionally OK, go ahead and try it out.

Take a few deep breaths, then gently bring your attention back into your hands and lift your hands off your body.

If you need to jot down any notes for yourself, take a moment to do so. Often, as with dreams, the details that might provide insights down the road can fade.

Check in to see how you feel physically, energetically, emotionally.

∽ • ∽

∞ Chapter Three ∞

Just Connect

Well, your toe bone connected to your foot bone
Your foot bone connected to your heel bone
Your heel bone connected to your ankle bone
Your ankle bone connected to your leg bone

Your leg bone connected to your knee bone
Your knee bone connected to your thigh bone
Your thigh bone connected to your hip bone
Your hip bone connected to your back bone

Your back bone connected to your shoulder bone
Your shoulder bone connected to your neck bone
Your neck bone connected to your head bone
I hear the word of the Lord!

I love this old song, because to me it is saying: if we address how all the parts connect, we are whole, and we can "hear the word of the Lord!" — we recognize spirit shining through us.

Early on in my training, my Councils said, "Disconnection equals pain. Connection equals pleasure and healing." They did not say this as an absolute dictum but, rather, in the context of trying to teach me about the concept they were calling "connection."

"Consider when you cut your finger," they said, "the separation of skin from its usual integration sends signals of pain to your brain. Even a simple paper cut can create sharp sensations of pain. Consider when you speak to a person and feel your spirit shared and returned. That is *connection*. When you try to speak to someone you love and they don't hear you, take you in, respond with love, that is *disconnection*, even if there is technically an exchange. And it is painful."

When your body or mind connects with something it loves — a person, an idea, an activity, a substance — energies flow, weave, and animate you. And you heal. When you disconnect from (or fail to connect with) your body, mind, or spirit, the alarm bells ring in the form of pain, symptoms, and dysfunction.

In this changing world, many of us have experienced both accelerated disconnections and new kinds of connections. Consider what months of isolation from pandemic shutdown, separating us from our life as usual, have done to our sense of the world, coupled with the myriad new connections we have been exposed to via the internet.

And as we grow into understanding new ways of connecting, repairing our personal weave, we can use this understanding to heal ourselves and the planet.

It is a cliché, but still generally true, to point out that our conventional medical system is still very partitioned. If you have a problem with your hip, the practitioner rarely looks at the whole interplay of bones in your body. And if you have a disease state in one organ, the specialist generally focuses on that organ, ignoring the nutrition, lifestyle, and other *connections* that play into the life of that organ.

Even the so-called holistic healers often fall into our culture's tendencies to want to drill down and identify a specific cause of the problem, so they can supply the missing chemical or eliminate the triggering agents, without taking into account the whole story of how your imbalance evolved and the interplay of factors that keeps it in place.

But healing ourselves and the planet involves awakening to this larger, more integrated kind of thinking that recognizes our interwoven nature. It asks us to learn to cultivate the web of connections that will nourish us, and it invites us to discover what it means to each of us, moment by moment, to connect with our own body, mind, spirit, and story.

When I am ailing or suffering or in pain, the first advice my Councils tend to give me is, "Just connect." And by that they mean: show up, turn off the spiraling mind, inhabit my body, and let myself connect back up to "dem bones" that form my inner structure. If I am willing to encounter the pain itself, it will show me where the tears in the fabric can be found and how to weave it back into connection. Reconnecting "dem bones" helps me to hear the voice of the Divine trying to express itself through me.

Protocol: Just Connect

It is tempting when you are struggling with pain to either (a) take a pill to try to get rid of it, (b) try to talk or rationalize yourself out of the pain, (c) try to ignore and push through the pain, or (d) try to deflect the discomfort, by reverting to a habit such as eating sugar, picking a fight, or overexercising.

Next time you are faced with pain, try this instead: No matter whether your pain is physical, emotional, or existential, bring your attention to your breath. Watch yourself breathe in and out, just tuning in to the sensations in your body, including any sensations of pain. Notice what shifts or moves, intensifies or lessens, as you breathe.

Then, when you are ready, follow these steps to tune in to and reconnect your chakras, or energy centers. (We will discuss chakras in depth in chapter 13.)

1. **Second and third chakra hold.** Place one hand on your second chakra, between the pubic bone and belly button (see figure 3.1). Place your other hand on your third chakra, at your solar plexus. If you do not have the use of your hands, ask someone to help you do the holds or to fasten a green tree leaf

over these areas. (Trees connect our three densities, the Earth Elemental Self, Talking Self, and Wiser Self!)

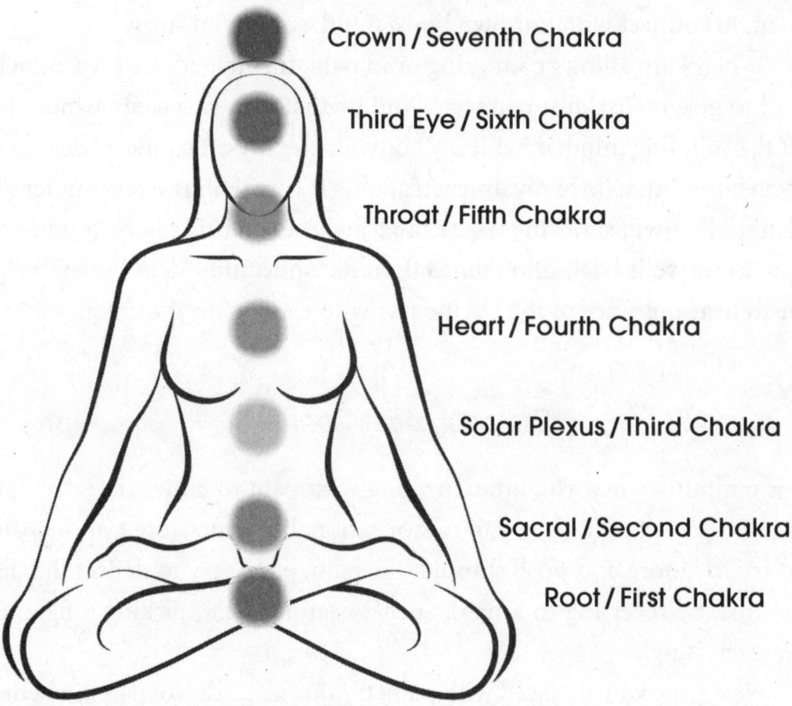

Crown / Seventh Chakra

Third Eye / Sixth Chakra

Throat / Fifth Chakra

Heart / Fourth Chakra

Solar Plexus / Third Chakra

Sacral / Second Chakra

Root / First Chakra

Figure 3.1. The seven chakras

Hold these two areas until you feel you are connecting in with each of them, *as if your hands can both hear and speak to the places on your body where they are sitting.*

Adapt these instructions to your particular situation. If you have the use of only one hand, move back and forth between the two areas. If touch is too painful, you can hold your hands slightly off your body and let the heat from your palms do the connecting.

This hold can take a while if you are not used to connecting in with your own body. Be patient as you tune in.

2. **Figure-eight between the second and third chakras.** Once you feel you have connected into your second and third chakras, figure-eight between them, either by moving one hand in a figure-eight motion, touching each chakra as it passes, or by sending an imaginary energetic figure eight looping between your two held areas. (Note: in Eden Energy Medicine, *figure-eighting*, used as a verb, signifies a gesture you make with your hand that sets your energies moving in a figure-eight pattern to support integration of your subtle energies and healing. Like stirring a pot, the motion is more than just tracing a shape; it actually gets energies moving the way they are supposed to move.)

3. **Third and fourth chakra hold.** When you feel that the figure eight has connected and is moving smoothly between your second and third chakras, keep one hand on your solar plexus and move the other hand up to cover your fourth chakra (heart chakra). Hold your heart chakra and solar plexus together until you feel your hands both speaking to and hearing those areas. Then figure-eight between the solar plexus and heart chakra, until the figure eight is smooth and comfortable.

4. **Fourth and sixth chakra hold.** Keeping one hand on your heart chakra, move your other hand to cover your forehead, over the sixth chakra (third eye). Hold your heart chakra and forehead until your hands are both speaking to and hearing those areas.

    Figure-eight between the two areas until you feel the figure eight moving on its own accord.

5. **Sixth and second chakra hold.** Finally, hold your hands on your forehead and your second chakra, just below your navel, until your hands are speaking to and hearing each area. Then hold a bit longer, until you feel them working in unison. It might feel like a gentle pulsing, or you might feel a figure eight forming between your two hands and moving smoothly. You might just get a thought in your head that they are now balanced. Figure-eight between these two chakras.

Tune in to the pain that sent you to this "Just Connect" protocol. Has it shifted in any way? How have your body, mind, emotions, thoughts, and spirit shifted during this time of "just connecting"?

Note: if you are not in the habit of connecting into your body's energies, you might find it easier to hold and tune in to each area individually first, then do the dual chakra holds as described above. Play with how to adapt these instructions for your own situation.

◌ • ◌

WHAT'S YOUR STORY?

Esther had a long list of ailments that depressed me when I heard it: she suffered from rheumatoid arthritis, her vision was degenerating, her feet had developed some kind of fungal infection, her mind was frequently foggy…and the litany went on and on. She found out about energy medicine online and was hoping it could help her.

I asked her what she was already doing to help herself, and her response was impressive. She was spending upward of two hours every morning meditating, using breathing exercises, and dutifully practicing a mishmosh of other techniques she had picked up in her search for relief. She was also following a healthy, but strict, diet prescribed by a nutritionist. But nothing seemed to work.

My heart went out to her. She truly wanted to find her way home to health. And in a way, she was pursuing the best advice she could find. But she was doing something I call "chasing monkeys."

Imagine you have dozens of monkeys you are keeping in a cage, and when you arrive to visit them, you discover the door is open and they are running crazed around your house. You try calling them, but they just look at you and laugh. You chase down one, then another, trying to corral them back into the cage. But each time you open the door to put a monkey in, another escapes, mocking you as it swings to freedom.

You can spend hours chasing down monkeys, exhausting yourself trying to contain them all again.

Or you can take a big, beautiful bunch of bananas, hang it in the cage, and holler, "Dinner's served." And watch the monkeys come running back home.

There are two ways to avoid chasing monkeys: (a) find the bananas that call the monkeys back home, and — perhaps more importantly — (b) stop keeping the monkeys in a cage at all. Instead, find a habitat where they will truly feel no need to escape.

Esther was following a vigorous regimen, doing everything she could think of to get better — except letting her body show her the bananas, moment by moment, that would help her energies to move and support her in finding joy, nourishment, comfort, and well-being. Her life was so centered around this disciplined healing regimen and the many things she believed she had to do in order to heal, she had no time to follow her inner guidance system and create the life she yearned for. Her intense self-help program created a stern and regimented cage and prevented her from building the appropriate habitat where her monkeys could live free and thrive.

I asked her, "What makes your heart sing?" At first, she couldn't answer. She couldn't name a single banana. She said that doing her daily exercises made her feel better, because they gave her hope. But they did not, in fact, seem to be improving her symptoms. And though she believed the food she was consuming was good for her, she had to force herself to eat it.

"If you could wave a magic wand and make it happen," I asked further, "is there anything that would make your heart sing?" She began to cry. "Dance," she said, "but I will never be able to do that again." And then she told me her story.

Esther's parents enrolled her in dance classes as a young girl because she was shy and had a slight stutter and they thought it would give her a way to communicate nonverbally. And their strategy worked beautifully. She loved dance, felt herself part of a community, got stronger, and even found herself more comfortable with speaking, as the dance helped her organize her thinking.

She danced all through her school years and then, once she began working, took evening or weekend classes just to keep dancing whenever she could. But in her early thirties she began to suffer one injury after another, and she gradually stopped enrolling in dance. She let the pressures of work and family shape her schedule. She told herself she was too old to dance anyway. By the time she was forty, she was diagnosed with rheumatoid arthritis and was told to avoid physically strenuous activity. Everything just snowballed downward from there.

At the root of all illness, disease, and dysfunction, there is a story or set of stories that frames how we interpret things, what choices we make, how we react both energetically and emotionally. That story acts as a habitat — often, as a cage — to keep us stuck in the same behaviors, reactivity, and stressors.

I am not just talking about a psychological story. Esther's history and present circumstances told an energy story. It showed us the weave of choices, interpretations, patterns, and movements of energies that gave her life and experiences meaning. By the time I met her, the story guiding Esther's life was all about illness, pain, breakdown, dysfunction, and the failure of discipline to help her.

Needless to say, it was not a story that made her heart sing.

It is too simplistic to say that Esther's loss of dance caused her illness. But what we can say is that Esther's story shaped her choices, influenced how she felt about her experience, shaped how she reacted biochemically and physiologically to life. The stressors built into her story acted like straws on the camel's back: they broke down her system so that it could not move blockages from her joints, could not fight off a fungal infection, could not clear her purpose stream (the liver meridian in Chinese medicine, introduced in chapter 9), which helps you fulfill your life purpose and feeds the physical eyes.

Esther's healing task was not just to tune in to find bananas, moment by moment, though that is a great start. It was also to recognize and revise the story that kept her monkeys living in a harsh and unfulfilling habitat. When you explore your stories, you can recognize the energy dynamics that you can then address with energy medicine and lifestyle medicine.

WORKING WITH YOUR STORY

Story is another specialized term my Councils introduced early in my training. In a way, it was like the concept of connection, but on steroids.

It referred to the interweave of our subtle energies and how they create both physical reality and meaning in life. And though they used the term to talk about recognizing our energy story, we can apply everything we know about story to understand the interweave of our subtle energies: it has characters, setting, plot, narrative thread, voice (point of view), and meaning or impact.

Characters include the self you are creating via your body, mind, and spirit, and the people who influence you in any way. Healing self and world involves recognizing your role in creating and reacting to the characters that people your reality. How you use your body moment by moment is greatly influenced by who you think you are, how other people see you, and the roles you believe you and others are playing vis-à-vis one another.

Setting includes the physical, mental, and emotional landscapes that influence your character and your physiology. Your creature self (Earth Elemental Self), your mind (Talking Self), and your spirit (Wiser Self) all have different settings that register within and influence your body. Where do your creature self, mind, and spirit habitually hang out?

Plot is the set of events you engage in, what happens when. When you get up in the morning, you choose certain activities and reject others, whether on the basis of your own inclinations or because of larger plot elements such as job, family, or duty to others. These events give your character a chance to evolve or cause you to get trapped in situations that don't allow you to flourish.

Narrative thread is the glue that holds a story together. It is the pull of the story itself as it unfurls and adds detail. It is the meaning that links otherwise separate events. If plot is "what happens," narrative thread brings in "why it happens and what it relates to."

Voice (point of view) is the perspective that chooses, shades, and controls your unfolding story. It addresses the question of who is telling the story, why they are telling it, and how reliable is the choice of details, perspective on events, and presentation of characters.

Meaning or impact is how the story affects you personally and also how it affects others in your sphere. Included in this is the notion of *why* you have chosen to tell this story rather than another.

1. Tell the story of a situation you want to understand and/or change. You can write the story out, talk it into a recorder, or tell it to a nonjudgmental friend while recording it, then transcribe it.

2. Without judging the story, go through and underline every word that seems to have some significance. Often the words that carry the story's energy stick out and tell us something about key energetic elements. For example:

    Esther's <u>parents enrolled her</u> in <u>dance classes</u> as a <u>young girl</u> because she was <u>shy</u> and had a <u>slight stutter</u> and they thought it would <u>give her a way</u> to <u>communicate nonverbally</u>. And their <u>strategy</u> worked beautifully. She <u>loved dance</u>, felt herself <u>part of a community</u>, <u>got stronger</u>, and even found herself <u>more comfortable with speaking</u>, as the dance helped her <u>organize her thinking</u>.

3. Make a list of your key words. What do they tell you about the themes in your story? Group similar themes together:

    Parents enrolled her — young girl — give her a way — strategy
    Slight stutter — shy — more comfortable with speaking — communicate nonverbally
    Part of a community
    Dance classes — loved dance — got stronger — organize her thinking

4. Explore the implications of these themes in your life and choices. A story, even a basic paragraph detailing the situation, often acts as a hologram for the energy dynamics that co-create the illness or life challenge you are investigating. By exploring implications, I'm not referring to conducting psychological analysis or uncovering hidden feelings. Instead, you are asking yourself, *How do these themes and energy issues play out for me?*

Esther's first cluster of themes — <u>parents</u>, <u>young girl</u>, <u>strategy</u> — implies that her parents were actively trying to find lifestyle choices that would help Esther to thrive and grow. The questions arise: Does Esther make these kinds of strategic choices for herself now? Is there a way that she didn't pick up the baton to parent herself with such strategic thinking?

Her second cluster — <u>stutter</u>, <u>shy</u>, <u>more comfortable with speaking</u>, <u>communicate nonverbally</u> — suggests that Esther's nature needs support to communicate. She needs to look at how well she communicates with herself and think about how to find situations that support her to communicate her essence, like dance did.

Her third cluster — <u>part of a community</u> — pointed to something Esther could explore: What did that community do for and to her? And did any present opportunities she had chosen make her feel the style of membership she loved?

The fourth cluster — <u>dance classes</u>, <u>loved dance</u>, <u>got stronger</u>, <u>organize her thinking</u> — raises the question: What could Esther do right now, in her present condition, that she loved and that would strengthen her? The two-hour daily routine she was pursuing was not a lovefest; it was a down payment on something she had been led to believe would yield returns. But that was not happening for her.

5. Take some time to look at each element of your story separately. Too often we jump to asking, "What does it mean?" and try to define the symbolic meaning of an event, illness, or conversation, rather than reflecting on its dynamics and impacts. Ask yourself the following questions:

    - Who are the *characters* in my story? What does each character want? What does each character contribute to the plot? Who belongs here, and who needs to be edited out?

    For Esther, characters included her younger self, her adult self, her parents, and perhaps dance itself or the dance community. And in her larger story, her many illnesses might be explored as a character, as well as her family and work.

- What is the *setting* and how does that influence what happens and how it happens in my story? What is missing in the setting? What needs to be changed or removed?

Esther was able to list what she loved about dance classes — the music and rhythm and feeling those in her body. She loved that the activities were organized and she just needed to sign up and participate. She liked the smells and sounds. She liked doing things with other people that weren't necessarily interactive. She liked getting to know people nonverbally. She came up with a better understanding of what dynamics of the setting were meaningful for her, which she could then look for in new contexts.

- What is the *plot* that gives this event or story context? Getting a rash is just an event. Getting a rash after visiting relatives, overworking in the yard, and watching a scary movie makes it a plot element. It might not point to cause and effect, but it may make the interweave of energies more apparent.

The most obvious plot in Esther's story was that she had dance at the center of her life, then gradually let it fall by the wayside, and finally was unable to do it because she was too sick. But subplots included watching her body break down and ascribing it to age, as well as her acceptance of other priorities crowding out her heart's desire. A third subplot was treating illness as the culprit and making a series of choices related to that, rather than seeing illness as a messenger and responding with choices to step in and parent herself with wiser strategies.

- What is the glue, the *narrative thread*, that makes this situation significant to you, as a narrator and character; to the other characters; and to the evolving story line? How does the narrative thread need to be altered or enhanced to make it more supportive of the story you wish to tell?

One narrative thread for Esther was the role of agency — how much others chose and decided for her versus what she chose and made happen for herself. Another thread was the role of love — her parents' love for her, her love of dance, and her dislike (failure to love) within her present circumstances. A narrative thread Esther recognized over time was the role of verbal versus nonverbal communication in how she felt membership and communion.

- What is the *voice* of this story? Who is telling it, how old are they, how much agency do they have in influencing the story? You can learn a lot from how a voice sounds when someone is speaking. What does the telling of this story show you about your own emotions and energetic participation in it? Who would you like to hear telling this story? (Sometimes, after I tell myself a story about some painful event I've experienced, I retell it in the voice of my Wiser Self, to see what I can learn from hearing it in a different voice.)

When Esther told her story to me, her voice alternated between a little girl's way of speaking — simple sentences, very direct — and a kind of clinical, objective voice, perhaps her work persona or the busy parent telling herself she no longer had leisure to indulge in activities like dance when she had obligations to others.

- What *meaning* did you assign to this event or set of events? What did it do for you literally and symbolically? If the impact affected you symbolically but not literally, do you choose that as the symbol that guides your body's chemistry and mind's framing at this time?

The meaning Esther assigned to the story was that she couldn't have what she wanted. Implied in this was that she didn't want what she had. So she needed to reframe that situation to see it as a death and rebirth: an opportunity to find something new to love rather than seeing herself irrevocably locked out from what could make her heart sing.

When you treat your story as a map of meaning, as a fabric of interwoven energies, you will deepen your recognition of the themes and dynamics that hold that fabric together. This perspective gives you more choices in what you weave into your life moving forward. If you are weaving in other people's definitions of your problems and other people's solutions, society's beliefs and interpretations, and groupthink understandings and reactions, you may want to reclaim authorship of your life. How can you rewrite your story — even the parts that are tragic, painful, and involve loss — with better developed characters, plot, narrative thread, voice, and assigned meanings?

Quick update on Esther: once she was able to recognize the energy themes that were blocking her, she found a number of ways to bring art and community back into her life. She organized a film series on dance from different cultures through her local library, which gave her ways to spend nonverbal time with like-minded others. She fell in love with learning about other traditions and volunteered at a nearby international institute to help visiting students adjusting to their new lives in her city. Supporting others who struggled to communicate strengthened her confidence. Her body stopped shouting at her, and her long list of ailments healed as she learned to find the bananas that were most nutritious for her.

RECONNECTING FROM THE INSIDE OUT, BOTTOM UP

Randy was in his midforties when he was stopped in his tracks, literally and figuratively. He prided himself on his discipline around staying in shape by working out at the gym three to four days a week. When people would praise him, he'd say, "Use it or lose it." His routine workouts included strength training on weight machines, as well as running or swimming. He considered himself in excellent shape.

One day, he was walking through the park just as a pickup game of soccer was forming. He'd played some soccer as a kid and loved it, so he decided on the spur of the moment to join the game. As he told me later, he looked the other players over and felt superior because he was probably in better shape than most of them: his weight was controlled, his muscles were well-defined, and he could still run and keep up without getting horribly winded.

However, about twenty minutes into the game, he noticed his body was aching from all the side-to-side, stop-and-start motions. And a few minutes after he decided to just push through the discomfort, he lunged for a ball and dislocated his knee.

He was lucky that his knee popped back into place, but he got himself to the ER for evaluation and followed the instructions to ice and brace it. He was diligent with his physical therapy and followed the guidance of his practitioners. Within record time, he was told that everything looked fine on the scans and he could slowly restart his former exercise program.

Only he couldn't. His body began letting him know, via pain and resistance, that something was not right. When he tried to get back into his gym routine, his knee was sore — that was to be expected. But sometimes his other knee would hurt, or his back would start aching, as if it too were injured. He would feel like he suddenly had a sprained ankle, and he frequently woke up with a sore neck. He was terrified he would lose his conditioning for good, so he plunged into a process of seeking help that included thousands of dollars' worth of consultations and treatments: not just medical scans, but scientific nutritional analysis and a strict diet, exercises to rebuild the muscles supporting his knee, thrice weekly chiropractic visits, even psychotherapy to deal with his frustration at being sidelined by injury.

After a few years of this, he showed up in my office, rather sheepish about seeking energy help (at the insistence of his sister). What jumped out at me about Randy's story was this: he was injured while trying to play, whereas his usual mindset about how to care for his body was to work out. His many therapies were aimed at rebalancing him so that he could return to his earlier way of being. And his body was making him chase monkeys with the wandering pain.

So how could Randy start to listen to his body, let it show him the way, partner with it, and get off the merry-go-round of therapeutic inputs? He, too, needed to find new bananas, but more importantly, he needed to reconnect with his body from the ground up, rather than subjecting it to ongoing therapy supplied by other people. The protocol below, "Restacking Your Boxes," helped Randy to work from the inside out and bottom up, and it cleared the persistent pain.

Why? Because for once Randy was assembling his parts into a balanced whole. But as he did it, something strange began to happen. His thinking and desires started to shift. First, he was just thrilled he could do something to fix himself, instead of having to run to a practitioner for adjustments. But then he started looking at his life and asking how to balance *those* boxes. And he began to see that he had always set goals and worked toward them, often pushing ahead like a bulldozer, rather than stopping to interact (play) with each box and build the balance from within.

This was also a key energy exercise (used together with finding bananas) that helped Esther re-sort her priorities and reset her body's weave of energies. Over the course of six months, this enabled her to clear most of her ailments.

Protocol: Restacking Your Boxes

Imagine your body is a lovely stack of boxes. I always picture gift boxes of different colors and shapes, with wonderful presents inside. Because the boxes are all different shapes and sizes, it's a little tricky to balance and stack them just right. It helps if you start at the bottom and build the column from the ground up.

With this energy exercise (like most in this book) I invite you to use your hands and gestures in combination with your imagination to restack the boxes as described below. While visualization can be helpful and contribute to the experience, subtle energies understand the communications of gesture, touch, movement, and actions even better. Therefore, let yourself play with this practice, the way a young child might throw a tea party for her teddy bears and actually go through the motions of setting the table, serving, buttering the scones, and sipping the tea.

The first time Randy experienced this in my office, when we worked together to restack his boxes one by one, he was amazed by how well his body responded to these subtle gestures, as if it were receiving actual chiropractic adjustments.

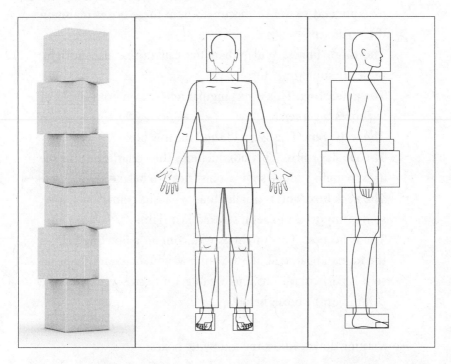

Figure 3.2. The segments of the body visualized as stacked boxes

The boxes I generally work with include:

- **The toe boxes.** I adjust each toe individually and get it to line up with the main box of the foot.
- **The foot boxes.** These need to rest squarely on the earth and have good balance relative to each other.
- **The ankle boxes (optional).** These are thin boxes, smaller than the size of the foot box they sit on. These often need some imaginary bubble wrap put in to cushion them.
- **The calf boxes.** These are tall and vertical, stretching from above the ankle to below the knee.

- **The knee boxes.** These are shorter than the calf boxes and square. They need to be placed well to connect the calf and thigh boxes and to hold their position when the body is moving. I also use hand motions to insert energetic bubble wrap or a pretend swivel connector to help these boxes maintain their balance.
- **The thigh boxes.** Wider than the calf boxes, also upright, these are sometimes top-heavy.
- **The pelvic box.** This is rectangular and sits on both stacks of leg boxes together.
- **The waist box.** This is a wide and narrow box.
- **The rib cage box.** This box includes the collarbone and the arms hanging down, so it is a bit tricky to balance.
- **The neck box.** This is smaller than what sits below and above, so it is important to get it stacked just right.
- **The head box.** This might as well contain a bowling ball — the human head is about the same weight, heft, and shape — so it is particularly challenging to get it to sit squarely on the column of the boxes below.

Now, sitting down, adjust the following boxes:

1. Starting with your toe boxes, you are going to grasp your big toe, either by holding the toe itself or by holding your fingers slightly away from the skin and grasping the energy box that contains your toe. Breathe in, and on the exhale, gently jiggle, twist, pull, or push your big toe so that it sits squarely and easily in relation to your foot box. You do not have to labor at this. Do it by feel; use your intuition. You are adjusting the toe with nudges and hints or even just with energetic shifts.

   Then proceed to rebalance the other toes on the same foot, one by one. Repeat the process on the other foot, until all your toes are square to your foot boxes and you feel the blood and energy flowing easily through them.

2. Then grasp either the sides of one foot or a slightly larger imaginary box encasing your foot. Breathe in, and on the exhale, jiggle and adjust your foot box until it is square to your leg — not twisted, tilted, torqued, or shoved too far forward or back. This is a gentle nudge, not a strong shove! Keep adjusting the box, letting your hands intuitively adjust your foot to get it in right relationship with your leg and with the other foot. When you set it down, it should sit solid and square on the earth but have flexibility and bounce from the arch. If the arch needs reshaping, use your hands and exhales to do that.

    Repeat this procedure for the other foot.

    Then adjust each ankle box the same way. If needed, slip some energetic padding in between each of these boxes to cushion them.

3. Stand up. Make sure the stacked toe, foot, and ankle boxes are secure and solid in the upright position, ready to handle the weight of the rest of the stack. If not, go back and reinforce these boxes as needed.

4. Adjust your calf boxes the same way. You may find it challenging to get just the right placement of the calf box relative to the ankle-foot base. Does it need to be twisted, moved forward or back, tilted on its axis? Grasp the calf, or the energy box containing it, and use your exhales to move it into perfect alignment to hold the rest of the stack. (Note: if your upper boxes are massively out of balance, you might need to adjust everything up to the hip box while continuing to sit.)

    Occasionally the boxes from the ankles up need to be lifted slightly, to allow you to reposition them on the stack. Use your intuition or the wisdom of your hands to feel what you need to do to get the stack balanced, just as you would do if you were working to rebalance a literal stack of boxes.

5. Adjust your knee boxes, inserting bubble wrap as needed. If these boxes twist and torque out of alignment, you may need to reinforce the strength of each box (adding energetic spacers can help) or put them on swivel platforms that allow

them to move independently of the boxes below and above. Remember to check all dimensions of balance, including forward or backward placement on the column you are creating.

6. Adjust your thigh boxes. You may need to use your hands to grasp and sway them back and forth or from side to side to balance them, since they are generally top-heavy. Make sure to balance them relative to each leg stack *and* to each other.

7. Adjust your pelvic box. This box may be the key to the strength of the whole stack. If it is tipped forward or back, the boxes above will be stressed, experience pain, and eventually tumble. If it is tipped side to side, the pressure will not be even on the two leg stacks, and the individual boxes will buckle over time.

8. Adjust your waist box. Most often, this is twisted to the right or left or shoved too far backward or forward. It is a small box but can tip the pile.

9. Adjust your rib box. I work with my hands on or near my rib cage, but often I have to adjust each arm to hang correctly, so it doesn't drag my rib box out of alignment.

10. Adjust your neck box. This is another key box in the stack. If it is too far forward or back, tipped or torqued, it not only can influence the balance of the box above it but can even have ripple effects down to the ankle box and foot box.

11. Adjust your head box so its considerable weight is held in place by being balanced on the stack of boxes rather than by the neck muscles.

CO • CD

An unbalanced stack creates pressures below and above the obvious mis-stacked box. So a pain in your hip or neck or side or any part of your body can in fact be a result of overall mis-stacking, rather than a problem with the painful joint or body part itself. That's what happened to Randy. His knee tissue healed, but his stack of boxes was not balanced.

Often an imbalanced stack will create a zigzag pattern of pressure, both physically and metaphorically. What I mean by a zigzag imbalance is a set of pressures on the skeleton that zigzag up the body, from side to side or front to back.

"Restacking Your Boxes" can improve the physical alignments of your muscular-skeletal system, but it also works energetically on your life, to give your Talking Self a more grounded, appropriate posture. Just as your story is a hologram for your subtle energies, your body is a hologram for the flow of energies within you. Connecting into each part and restacking your boxes as needed brings greater stability and unity to your ongoing creation of self.

⌒ Chapter Four ⌒

Beyond Binary

I have always been a miserable failure with true/false and multiple choice tests! As I read the questions, my mind starts to create circumstances where each answer could be true. And even when I know which answer they are looking for, I want to argue with the creators of the test, to show them how none of their answers is perfect and all of the possible answers have merit.

At one point, this habit caused me to fail at math. I was taking a test and got utterly stuck on a question about a farmer with six fingers on each hand who was counting his sheep. The question was, if he said he had 347 sheep, how many did he really have? I didn't care how many sheep he had. Presumably he was far beyond counting on his fingers. I had other questions: How did having twelve fingers affect his life? Did he have trouble dating? Did other kids make fun of him and cause him to become a sheep farmer to get away from their judgments? I couldn't finish the test because the original question pulled me into another world.

It must have driven the adults in my life crazy to have me constantly trying to explain all the possibilities. But now I suspect it was good preparation for the empowered yin thinking that is moving into our shared consciousness.

The yang era that is moving out has been characterized by *contrast* — binary concepts of good versus evil, us versus them, true versus false. As we experience the last gasps of patriarchy, these binaries are intensifying. The world seems to be determined to break into opposing camps and stop listening to the "other side."

Contrast is when we know something by what we compare it to: the notion that we learn our lessons through adversity, decide what to do on the basis of the most pressing problems or crises, then compete to get individual glory or privilege that allows us to rise above the fray.

A non-contrast view says we all have something to contribute to the weave of life. Our best motivation comes, not from competing, but from successful collaborations and using our very individual gifts to support our shared reality.

A contrast view of illness is that we have the wrong inputs, or didn't take care of ourselves, or inherited bad genes; and now we need to find perfect inputs or the magic treatment that will torpedo the illness and liberate us to be well.

A non-contrast view of illness is that we all have areas where our energies are flowing and interacting and others where they are clogged or diverted. We are well and sick and everything in between. If we dip below a threshold of health, we are not looking to find the magic inputs or treatments; we are looking to shift how our energies move and interact and express themselves physically, mentally, spiritually. Cultivating well-being is something we do in an ongoing way, on behalf of ourselves *and* the larger weave of life-forms.

If you are sick, how are you also well? And what lies in the territory between sick and well? More importantly: How does the energy of *contrast* — comparing yourself to others, judging your experience, interpreting it in binaries of good/bad, us/them, and perfect/flawed — pile on straws that are breaking your camel's back?

∽ Play with It! ∽

Take a few moments to make a list of all the straws on your camel's back —
all the stresses, obligations, duties, and demands and also the self-chosen
goals, aspirations, and expectations. When you get up in the morning and
start your day, to what extent are you encountering a blank slate or a simple aspiration? To what extent do you encounter instead your list of what
needs to happen, what is wrong, what must be fixed?

Sort your list by grouping the "straws" into categories. What are the
categories your mind comes up with?

If they are rooted in good/bad, pleasure/duty, or other binaries, ask
yourself how each task on your list can contribute to your well-being, to
the larger weave of life-forms, to the health of the planet, and to the quality of your lived experience today.

With each item, ask yourself what would happen if you just dropped
it from the list.

If your list is judgmental or binary, be kind to yourself. Do some of
the other exercises in this chapter to help you shift away from either/or
thinking.

∽ • ∽

The yang culture that is moving out was built around the "hero's journey" — the story of someone who overcomes tremendous adversity to
win the girl or boy, earn the money, magically heal some incurable disease,
break free from oppression. I have had hundreds of clients who were addicted to contrast, to drama, and to adrenaline, which contrast stimulates.
These clients, without always realizing it, somehow needed to create problems or illnesses so they could get their gratification when they solved or
healed them. I say this without blame. It's a cultural obsession — and I've
been there myself!

Who doesn't love a good superhero, miracle cure, viral social media post,
scandal, breakout performance in a competition, or squirt of adrenaline?

However, part of the radical change of this time is that we are now
being asked, individually and collectively, to move from binary either/or
thinking to awareness of the full circle of possibility. Maybe *The Lion King*

was a foreshadowing! We are being asked by the earth herself to partici-pate in the full circle of life.

We are being pushed by phenomena such as global warming and the Covid-19 pandemic to shift our thinking, choices, and even our biochem-istry to create a world where the collective weave is more valued than the contrast. A world where individual gain does not trump collective good and where these two poles are not either/or choices but part of a whole range of possibilities that are right in their own time. We are being asked to stop glorifying the negative teachers of adversity, struggle, suffering, and threat (though we can still address these challenges and meet them with compassion) and instead start to embrace and value positive teachers from whom we can learn new ways of being.

This does not mean that we jettison our respect for someone who overcomes difficulties. That is part of being human. But it is not the es-sence of what gives this life meaning.

Stephen Hawking always comes to my mind in this respect. He was a brilliant cosmologist and theoretical physicist who lived for fifty-five years with ALS, a degenerative disease. You can see his life as a hero's journey of overcoming adversity to accomplish great things. Or you can see his life as rich and full of accomplishments in science and see him as someone with a disability who was skillful in transacting life, as a thinker about the nature of life itself, and as a sometimes successful, sometimes inadequate father, friend, teacher, and husband.

Instead of defining him as amazing because of the contrast and the adversity he lived with, we can define him as amazing because of his multiplicity and contributions and the sheer extent of humanity he ex-plored. His self-chosen epitaph was not "He accomplished great things despite or because of his disability." It was his most famed contribution: the Bekenstein–Hawking entropy equation.

POSITIVE TEACHERS

I once asked my Councils, "What is the purpose of life on planet earth?" They answered, "Increase." As I have mentioned, they often use vocabu-lary in very specialized ways. A word for them is like a crystal reflecting many dimensions of understanding. "Increase," they explained, "is when the soul comes into embodiment to enrich itself through lived experience. What you live and choose and embody here enriches your soul, just as your soul feeds you energetically in specific ways and funds certain choices more than others."

I've never been a big fan of the term *downloading*, in part because for me it lacks this crystalline structure. The nature of guidance, in my experience, is not like downloading material, or taking dictation, or getting instructions. It is more about creating a connection with a source of wisdom and learning from it. It is an energetic exchange — often a multidimensional exchange that happens through my mind, heart, gut, and body and resonates throughout my life and story line — not just a one-way transmission. It is an exchange that supports increase.

My Councils were forever introducing me to *positive teachers*, sources of wisdom, often found in the natural world, and suggesting that cultivating well-being (whether you are sick or just interested in evolving) happens when you link to positive teachers and let your mind and energies entrain to the energy structures they offer.

The word *entrain* originally meant "board a train." But it is used now in many fields to describe the phenomenon of connecting up to something that pulls you into its sphere and moves you forward.

I had to relearn this lesson of entraining to positive teachers the hard way in 2020, when I got addicted to listening to news, painting a very binary narrative of events, and framing our world as a struggle between good and evil. These stories, while rooted in true events, were drains on my energy, pulling me into binary thinking (entraining me) and causing me stress up the yin-yang!

Although I know tons of energy medicine exercises, it was returning to some of the basic teachers, breath and walking, that best helped me rebalance my energies.

Guided Visit: Breath Is Your Teacher

Spend a few minutes just watching your breath, without trying to influence it or control it. Is it deep and easy, or do you stop yourself on the inhale, cut off the part where your body is using the oxygen, release only partway, or rush into the next breath?

Just notice which part of the motion is smooth and which part is challenged. This can actually give you a lot of insight into how you transact with energies across the board.

Notice when your breath is moving in, and when it is moving out…

Now, notice all the points within "in" and "out"…filling, filling, filling, pausing when full, then turning, emptying, emptying, releasing, letting your lungs deflate, and resting empty.

Experiment with moving your hand in concert with your breath. Correlate the gesture with an inhale, then an exhale, and then let your hand move through the whole circle of in and out and everything in between. What happens when you correlate physical movement with your breath?

Breath can help to move energy. Inhaling often brings the energy in or activates it; exhaling often helps to power a shift or guide a release. But the whole cycle of breathing alters your body and mind in myriad subtle ways. Tune in and see what moves and shifts as you breathe.

Find a place on your body where you are experiencing pain or tightness. Putting one hand there to guide your attention, send your breath into the area. Experiment with whether it wants the inhale or the exhale energy, both, or some particular part of the breath cycle.

Just hold this area through several inhales and exhales, noticing what happens there and throughout your body.

You might want to ask the Universal Supply Center for some energetic medicine to add to the breath: love, forgiveness, compassion, or even an energetic painkiller. All medicine is a form of messaging. The breath, fascia, blood, bones, and water are all excellent carriers of energetic messaging.

Experiment with two breath patterns: (a) inhale peace, exhale stress; and (b) inhale stress, exhale peace. What happens in your body as you experience these two patterns?

Both can help you move toward peace and release. Practice one of these patterns for several minutes, then stop to investigate whether the pain has shifted.

∽ • ∽

WALKING IS YOUR TEACHER

I went through a phase in my training with the Councils when I would get caught up in too many emotions. It was as if all the energy work I was doing stirred up the dust bunnies, and my inner world was full of swirling feelings and sensations and thoughts. Invariably, my Councils would say, "Go walk." For a while I thought they were just asking me to blow off steam, change my environment.

But they weren't saying, "Go for a walk." They meant that the activity of walking was going to give me the energy shift that I needed.

"Walk" meant using my body to move past stuck energies.

When you walk, your foot first lifts from the earth. It leaps into the void as it swings forward. Then it lowers, connects with the earth (even on an inside surface while you are wearing shoes), sets in place, shifts weight, and pumps what I used to call earth juice up from the planet.

To me, walking feels like I am fueling my body and also aligning it with the wisdom of the planet itself as I step down, feel the weight, feel my ankle bend, shift my weight forward, send my other foot out into the unknown, then watch that foot lower, plant, roll forward, shift weight, and pump up earth juice. And the left/right motion helps support my left and right brains to cross over and communicate better.

Although there are binaries within walking — lift/set, left/right — as there are within breathing, there is so much more going on. Walking is quite magical, energetically speaking. We are being fed by the earth. We are pumping that energy up into our body. It feeds and stimulates various distributors in our energies and revitalizes the energy streams that are called *meridians* in Chinese medicine.

But more is happening there as well. Your foot has radar in it that communicates with all the life-forms on the planet (see "Balancing Your Sonar Rings," page 267). Walking helps activate and bring that communication into many centers in your body that can use and respond to the information.

Your blood gets stimulated with a rhythm that shifts and balances how it communicates.

The water that comprises most of your makeup becomes tidal (think of water sloshing in a glass as you walk), moving in rhythms that echo the rhythms of the earth.

The bones compress and release in patterns that strengthen them.

The lymph, which cleans and clears toxins, gets pumped and supported in its work.

Try this: for a day or two, every time you feel your energy, thoughts, or emotions clog up or falter, walk with this kind of attention for a few minutes, preferably outdoors, but indoors is fine. What happens to your body, to your breathing, to your mind, to your emotions, and to your perspectives?

It is no accident that many spiritual traditions include breath work and walking meditation. Both are energetic treasure troves that act as powerful teachers, powerful medicine.

If you have difficulties with breathing or walking, explore ways you can entrain to these teachers differently. One client who had horrible problems with asthma and breathing found that if she put one hand on her partner's lungs and the other on her own, then let her body entrain with her partner's lungs, after some time her own lungs would learn from her partner's body and reset their cadence.

Mothers use this phenomenon all the time with infants, particularly those who were born prematurely. Placing your infant on your chest not only entrains and teaches your infant to breathe, it actually strengthens their resilience. In parts of Africa, where mothers within traditional cultures typically carry their infants on their chests or backs most of the time, crib death is practically nonexistent.

Another client who broke both legs in a fall could feel her whole body becoming out of whack from her inactivity and inability to walk. She explored sitting on the earth and kneading the ground as if her hands were walking, and she could feel her whole body responding to it. When her casts were removed, she was stunned to discover her leg muscles were far less atrophied than her doctor had warned her to expect.

This notion of entraining goes beyond learning intellectual concepts from a teacher or using the teacher as a role model. It means you enter their sphere of being, their worldview, their story. And it changes you, in myriad ways.

Exercise: Let the Earth Breathe You

Lie down on the earth with your chest downward, as if the earth is your mother and you are a baby being held against her heart. Feel your heart connect with the heart of the earth.

Send all your worries, pain, troubles, fears, tensions into the earth for storage or disposal.

Then send your hopes and dreams down into the earth, to plant seeds.

When you feel your heart beating in sync with the heart of the earth, roll over onto your back.

Now feel how the earth has your back, supporting each vertebra, holding you with her bulk and density and solidity. Let your weight sink into the earth; let her hold you. And listen or feel for the breath of the planet. You may not be able to consciously feel or hear this rhythm. But just let go of trying to control your own breathing and allow it to entrain to the breath of the planet. *Let the earth breathe you.* Let the earth breathe you, as the baby lets the mother guide her breathing into stronger patterns of inhale, pause, exhale, and rest.

You can just dwell in this activity for a while or proceed to let go of any thoughts and *let the earth think you.* Entrain to the mind of the planet and rest in its larger rhythms.

Then, when you are ready, bring your conscious thinking mind back on board and tune in to your own conscious breathing. Thank the mother for her wisdom and support. Stretch your limbs, yawn, blink your eyes, touch your arms or legs — bring yourself back to full body awareness — then get up and move on with your day, retaining a sense of entrainment to the earth and her rhythms.

⌘ • ⌘

NUMBERS ARE YOUR TEACHERS

Although I did fail math class in eleventh grade, I actually feel a deep affinity to numbers, and I use them as energy medicine. My father had savant syndrome, which meant he was extremely gifted in mathematical calculating and significantly less gifted in other realms (emotional intelligence, for example). I suspect my love of the energies of numbers is a kind of shadow syndrome, inherited from him.

I noticed at some point early on that when I would feel insecure or upset, I'd start counting or doing math problems in my head. I might review my budget, or figure out measurements, or count occurrences of various sorts to compare them numerically. Doing this would calm me, reset my energies, organize my chaotic feelings, even ground me.

To me, numbers carry energy and have something to do with an underlying energy architecture I don't yet fully understand. They influence my body, mind, and spirit. I've had dozens of clients ask their guides what the significance of 11:11 or 4:44 or 5:55 is on the clock. The answer is invariably that numbers can move and organize energies; repetitive numbers invoke balance.

My Councils used to talk about people being "ones, twos, or threes." What they meant by that was:

- Some people reference only their own inner truth, inner motivations, sourcing — the *ones.*
- Some people thrive on harmony and exchange with another — the *twos.*
- Other people thrive on discord, challenge, or change — the *threes.*

These numbers represent very different approaches to what people seek in terms of comfort and grounding.

I found this paradigm extremely useful in helping me to understand a person's behaviors and choices. I'd ask myself, *Is this person being a one, two, or three in this moment?* This basic one-two-three differentiation illuminated a lot of people's motivations for me.

For a one, separating from others to hear their own rhythm is their natural way to balance, not a sign of some kind of avoidance or dysfunction.

For a two, balance means learning to harmonize with specific people and activities and ideas that frame their life. When a two is distraught, they *need* to create harmony or agreement with another person, often even more than they need to be right.

For a three, balance means learning to create the right kind and amount of discord or challenge to promote growth. They are often energized by discord and enlivened by imbalance and change.

I'm not trying to divide people into strict categories and say they are always a one, two, or three. Rather, it is useful to ask: *In this moment, is this person operating as a one, two, or three, energetically?*

Self-fueling (one), harmonizing (two), and triggering challenge and change (three) are very different goals. If I don't know this, my need to stimulate change (three) might conflict with my partner's need to patch up an argument at all costs (two). Similarly, someone who loves to discuss and dispute (three) can't understand a partner who withdraws to go inward and refuel (one).

Needless to say, we often choose partners whose baseline habitual number is different from our own!

⚭ Play with It! ⚭

Bring to mind a recent event that knocked you off-balance. At that time, were you responding as a one, two, or three? Now, look at what happened in that event for you. Did it allow you to draw apart, if you were in a one phase? Did it allow you to harmonize, if you were in a two phase? Did it allow you to challenge others or the situation, if you were in a three phase?

Just play with the one, two, and three concept a bit. What number would you think the other person or people were operating from? How could you have asserted your need in that moment to do justice to your one, two, or three nature?

⚭ • ⚭

Numbers codify energetic insights in lots of spiritual traditions and energy taxonomies, including Kabbalah, tarot, numerology, astrology, medicine wheels, and more. In the years since my Councils first introduced that concept, I've played with combinations of twos and threes (harmony and disharmony) and evolved my own symbolic meanings for numbers four through ten:

- A *four* finds meaning not just in coupling, but in creating structures (two twos teaming up).
- A *five* finds satisfaction by helping things fall apart so they can reformulate (a combination of a three and a two).
- A *six* will often find fulfillment in collective action (three twos teaming up).
- A *seven* will find balance by following processes and completing cycles (the harmony of two, discord and change brought by three, followed by the harmony of two again).
- An *eight* will find meaning by participating and moving on, with the emphasis on movement (the march of two, two, two, two).
- A *nine* will find harmony only when nearing completion of a task after much struggle and challenge (created by the three threes built into their nature).
- A *ten* finds balance in trying to be the complete package, living every aspect of their experience and then reaping the rewards (two plus three, repeated twice).

Of course, if you are at all mathematical, you might be saying, "Yes, but eight can also be a three plus a two plus a three" — and that is true. This is not so much about math as it is about the fact that numbers speak to me to show me patterns of energy. If someone is seeking to heal, it is helpful to look at what pattern of energy they are operating under. What would evolution look like for a six? Moving into seven! And ten evolves by returning to one.

Though I can't claim a thorough knowledge of the inner architecture that's at work, I have observed an evolution of energy numbers: one brings the energy in, two harmonizes it, three sets it in motion to grow further, four stabilizes it into form, five allows it to break apart to support growth, six brings in collaboration, seven introduces cycles, eight shows a path forward, nine represents struggle leading to something larger, and ten brings it into a larger arena.

⟳ Play with It Some More! ⟲

Take the same situation and people you looked at before using one, two, and three. This time, ask yourself what number each person, including you, was expressing energetically, based on the descriptions of one through ten above.

What could you have done to support your own energetic phase in that moment? What could you have done to support or honor the energetic numbers each other person seemed to want or need?

This is a great tool to use for insight when you find yourself getting tangled in the verbiage and data of a situation. However, you can also use it as an energy medicine tool to shift energies.

Go back to the thought of the recent event. What number were you? Keeping the event in mind, use your hands to drum on your body, in a rhythm guided by that number. Or direct an imaginary orchestra to that time signature. Or walk that number of steps, then turn and repeat. Or bounce a ball that number of times, pause, and repeat.

Now, consider: what number did you *need* in that moment?

If, for example, you needed an eight — support in moving on — drum on your body or gesture or move to a rhythm of eight, then pause, and do it again, and pause, and repeat.

If we speak energetic numbers to the body, it responds by releasing the stress from a story line and moving to a more balanced state.

⟳ • ⟲

THE PLANET IS YOUR TEACHER

Many voices are speaking out on behalf of the planet right now, calling attention to the importance of saving her, of changing our ways, of conserving and protecting and understanding her better.

There is nothing like a global pandemic to wake people up to our inter-connectedness on this planet!

The thing is, we are not separate from the planet: we are part of her. So in saving the climate, and learning to use renewable resources, and learning to stop burning fossil fuels, we are learning to care for and heal ourselves. And by caring for ourselves we are saving the planet.

A *lot* of the illness that individuals experience arises from our collective failure to recognize our interrelationships and energetic exchanges with all life-forms on this planet. This goes beyond the obvious issues: the malnourishment from foods that no longer carry nutrients, the illnesses that arise from pumping substances into our shared air space that aren't meant for human or creature consumption.

Our refusal to see that we are part of the collective whole allows us to act in ways that rebound on our own health, our own well-being.

We have much to learn from the planet, and when I use the term *learn* I am not referring to intellectual insights or ideas. I'm talking about the process of letting our energies entrain with the planet and allowing it to influence us in multiple ways.

I am not alone when I confess to frequently falling out of harmony with cycles of light and dark. I don't rise with the sun and rest when it sets. Instead, I read books on my Kindle and use electric lights to create whatever illumination I want moment by moment. I guess I can't complain if I suffer eyestrain and my vision is myopic!

And I will confess that though I more or less pay attention to what time of year it is, I live in California, where the differences are subtle and it is easy to ignore the seasons that are meant to help regulate my body. So I can't be surprised if my ability to balance my body's temperature has been iffy at best. And this causes my adrenals and thyroid and blood sugar metabolism to have to work harder. It makes sense that I've had to address issues with my earth element (digestion, weight control) and my fire element (adrenals, energy rushes and crashes).

In our culture, we have been taught to see ourselves as a species apart from the earth. And because of that, we have deprived ourselves of our greatest energy medicine. As a kid who spent my childhood reading, preferably in bed under the covers, I had to make a conscious effort to get out and experience nature, love this earth, listen to her, and, most importantly, entrain to her and learn!

My greatest earthy teachers have been rocks, grass, cats, and dogs. I'm crazy about all of them. If I sit in the grass, I can feel the inter-connection of life-forms. I can feel the separate blades and the collective root system. And I feel renewed.

That is true when I hold a rock. Its solidity renews me.

And cats and dogs — they absolutely reset my heart and delight my soul and heal my hurt ego. And make me sneeze, a form of gatekeeper (immune system) release.

So although I can get overwhelmed by all the ways I'm not a nature child, I have learned that each time I interact with something natural, it does something to heal and reset my own body's rhythms. And it also allows me to rejoin the community of larger energetic exchanges.

Every life-form communicates with the larger weave of life-forms energetically, via light, sound, vibrations, and/or telepathy.

Scientists are rapidly identifying some of these natural communication networks. Have you seen the 2019 documentary *Fantastic Fungi*? It is amazing to see that the fungal realm has a visible communication web called the mycelium. Trees, too, though they appear separate, are able to share resources and information via their root systems and using the mycelium. Even bees, whales, wolves, and other creatures all have similarly subtle and fascinating inter-connections.

And that's the point. We do too. Not just the linkages we create through the World Wide Web, but energetic connectors among members of our species and energetic connectors between our species and others.

Part of the binary experiment in the yang era was to flatten our perceptions down to what could be described with words and ideas, causing us to ignore those energetic connections. This whole long yang-era experiment was an exercise in souls coming into this earthly dimension and putting on blinders, so they couldn't remember their root systems, their spiritual aspects, their inter-connectedness. Yet there is bleed through from those dimensions, and historically, individuals who saw the larger energetics of this world did not always fare well. Those who were wise in earth magic, particularly women and indigenous people, were often put to death for daring to recognize their inter-connectedness with all of life.

So now the blinders are slipping, and opening, and even dissolving, and many individuals are recognizing larger patterns and connections. They are recognizing influences beyond direct cause and effect. And our tools for healing and transforming our reality are growing exponentially.

It can seem like a huge job, to heal damaged bodies and minds, to change our habits and behaviors, to clean up our act when it comes to being part of a collective reality. But it's not: the universe is full of holograms, full of specific actions and connections and energy medicine, that will heal you and make you whole.

It starts with being willing to transcend binary thinking and really question *all* of the supposed opposites:

- Are savory and sweet really opposites? Or are they just flavors in a whole realm of possibility?
- Are dark and light opposites, or are they gradations on a circle of illumination that includes these two points?
- Are male and female opposites, or are they merely two socially assigned categories within a whole array of possible expressions of gender?

As I've mentioned before, our socialized minds have been trained to think in binary either/or terms. And what is erupting into our collective consciousness now is a recognition that those so-called opposites are not really binary at all. They are culturally assigned meanings that flatten our understanding into limiting either/or options.

If I think in terms of a flavor being savory or sweet and ask myself if I'm craving a savory or a sweet, I miss the myriad of choices and flavor perceptions that create a whole nuanced world of experience beyond those two categories.

Most people would say dark and light are opposites and belong at the far ends of a spectrum. We are taught to think that way. Yet in a twenty-four-hour cycle, light grows and grows until it turns, and then darkness grows and grows. Between the two assigned opposites, there are points of growing light and waning light, growing darkness and waning darkness.

If you see dark and light in nonbinary terms, they are two points on a circle that is characterized by gradual change. And that circle is part of a sphere that experiences most aspects of dark and light and everything in between, depending on where you stand!

Imagine that you live in a culture that is not so interested in absolutes but instead values nuance. That culture might speak in terms of waning and waxing moments, not darkest and lightest. Instead of declaring, "It's always darkest before the dawn," that culture might have a saying like "Life is seen best when the light shifts."

The binaries of our world, of our thinking, are breaking apart as consciousness rises.

Take the categories of male and female. You may have noticed that more and more young people in these changing times are declaring themselves to be nonbinary, neither male nor female. Our cultural logic would say: test the chromosomes to see what "they" really are. But X and Y are culturally assigned opposites. The science itself is still binary in its thinking.

Almost thirty years ago, my Councils told me that a new chromosome would be emerging: the Z chromosome. It would be neither male nor female, and I'd see it increasingly in clients who would be shifting away from these traditional identities in response to an inner makeup that did not fit the binary gender roles or understandings.

I don't know if science has discovered this yet. But the cultural evidence is there in how young people are experiencing and expressing a fuller spectrum of gender identification. I have worked with hundreds of clients who appear to have a strong amount of Z in their makeup, which is neither male nor female, and they struggle to understand their physicality, inner truth, and identity in a world that is so determinedly binary.

The reason this is relevant, beyond the humanity of letting our young people morph and create new definitions of what it means to be human, is that we tend to think of healing as getting "balanced," and we tend to think of balance as binary. "I have too much of this, so I need more of that."

When you add in a third chromosome, a third dimension, it shifts how you think about everything. Instead of "this" versus "that," you find yourself combining them with other ingredients: shared, partially shared, more or less separate, somewhat here, occupying multiple spaces, sometimes relevant, and so on. You bring in awareness of a spectrum that is not a line with binaries assigned to each end, but a circle, with positions that relate to one another in multiple ways.

Take a look at figure 4.1. A line is like the spectrum that spans light/dark, sweet/savory, or female/male. If that line rotates, it forms a circle of possibilities, or in many cases it depicts a cycle, like all the phases of the moon. And if you allow that circle to rotate on an axis, it becomes a sphere, a whole world of possibilities.

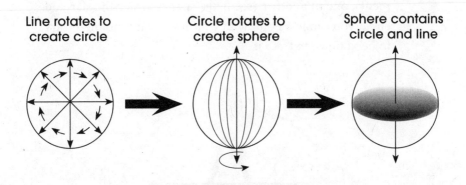

Line rotates to create circle   **Circle rotates to create sphere**   **Sphere contains circle and line**

Figure 4.1. From line to circle to sphere

Whatever you experience on one point of that sphere — or this earth — another experience of it is happening differently on another part of that sphere. The line and circle don't disappear; binary and linear and even cyclical experiences still exist. But they take on new meaning in the context of global, spherical consciousness.

Binaries are part of our sacred geometry, so we don't need to reject them completely: so-called opposites like yin and yang can be relevant to address. But traditionally yin and yang were wisely portrayed as part of a circle, with a drop of light in the center of the darkness and a drop of darkness in the center of the light. Our deeply felt sacred geometry is rooted in the *circle of possibilities* that modulate all those binaries and the *sphere* that is our home planet and source of the energies that feed us.

As we learn to use our *spheric consciousness*, rooted in our understanding of a more inter-connected world, we can heal ourselves and our planet in deeper, more influential ways. Here is an energy exercise that helps you anchor your energies in spheric consciousness.

Protocol: Anchoring in the Stabilizing Sphere

1. Stand where you have at least an arm's length of space around you. Trace a five-pointed star on the floor, representing the five elements of Chinese medicine (and other traditions), and draw a circle around it, representing the flow of those elements, one to another (see figure 4.2). To trace the star and circle, you can just point with your fingers; it is not necessary to bend down to trace it.

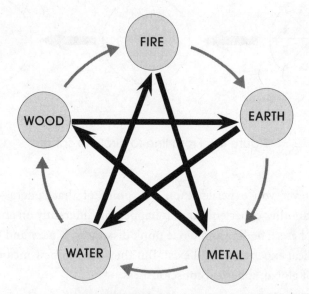

Figure 4.2. Draw a five-pointed star, starting with water, then a clockwise circle around it

2. Stand in the center of that star. Use your hands to trace a sphere around your body, at arm's length, around your front and back (like longitudinal lines) and create your sphere (see figure 4.3).

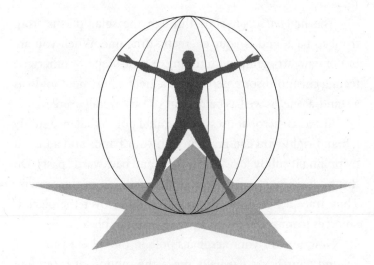

Figure 4.3. Stand in the center of your star
and trace a sphere around you

3. Now you are going to balance the two axis poles that co-create your sphere: the horizontal acrobat's pole and the vertical torus pole (see figure 4.4).

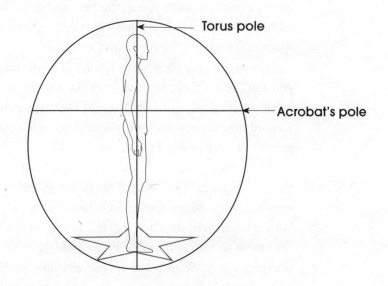

Figure 4.4. Acrobat's Pole and Torus Pole

The *acrobat's pole* runs through the solar plexus from front to back and is your energetic time line. When you are out of sync, struggling with timing or time usage, or otherwise feeling chrono-disoriented, this is a great adjustment to do as a stand-alone, as well as being part of this overall exercise.

Just as an acrobat uses a horizontal pole to balance subtly left and right, you can grasp it with your hands and adjust it by pulling it subtly forward (future) and backward (past). Do this by feel until you sense you are anchored in the present. Then trace a five-pointed star and a circle over the place it emerges from your solar plexus, to seal it in place.

Now, anchor your acrobat's pole in the sphere you drew around your body. I usually make the motion of extending it in each direction to plug it into the sphere in front of and behind me. I feel or imagine it clicking into place.

4. The *torus pole* is your energetic axis of place. It reminds me of the axis around which the earth turns, although it is not angled. It runs vertically through the center of your body, from above your head, through the base of your torso, and down into the earth. It keeps you in the here and now. You can readjust this pole whenever you experience disorientation in space or struggle to "be here now."

    Grasp the pole above your head and below your root (if you can't reach both, just use one). As you did with the acrobat's pole, gently and subtly adjust the torus pole. Move it upward and downward until you feel you are centered and present in your physical place.

    Trace the five-element star on the top of your head to seal the pole in place. Then extend the pole top and bottom and plug it in your sphere above and below you.

5. Now, stretch your arms and legs out in two wide V's and anchor them in your sphere (see figure 4.5).

6. Energetically hook into the sphere anything with twos on or in your body: eyes, ears, the chambers of your bicameral brain, shoulders, lungs, breasts, kidneys/adrenals, elbows, hips, knees.

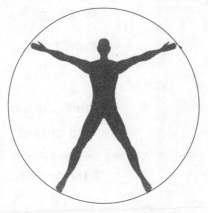

**Figure 4.5. Anchor your arms
and legs into your stabilizing
sphere**

7. Link in anything else on your body that needs to be connected. I often hook in my tailbone, my nose, and the point at the base of my skull, where it joins to the top of my neck.

8. Hook your first through seventh chakras — one at a time, front and back — into the sphere. Your seventh chakra extends upward; your first chakra extends both downward and outward. Your second through sixth chakras extend forward and back from the spine (see figure 4.6).

9. If you wish, you can also hook your worries or challenges into the sphere, to bring you more global perspective on them.

10. Infuse your sphere with whatever resources you feel will bring you more stability. You can use qualities, such as grace; positive teachers you admire; colors or sounds; and your daily gifts from your sniffer dog!

This exercise activates and anchors your spheric consciousness and helps you transcend linear, binary thinking. It also supports an energetic torus around you (see figure 4.7), reinforcing the natural waterfall circulation of your energies through your body and energy field.

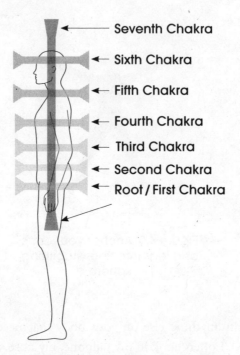

Figure 4.6. First through sixth chakras
extend both forward and back from the spine

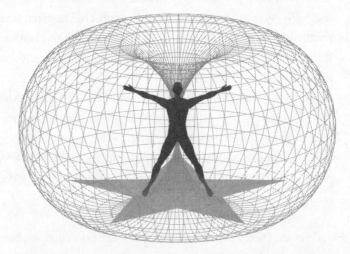

Figure 4.7. The torus of energies circulating through
and around your body

� • 98�

⚭ Chapter Five ⚭

Keeping the Gates of Self

In 2021, when air travel started to open up after the Covid-19 pandemic shutdown, airlines reported greatly increased incidents of aggression, hostility, and violence on the part of passengers. A Southwest Airlines flight attendant asked a woman to honor the mask requirement then in place, and the passenger hauled off and slugged her, breaking two teeth and bloodying her eye.

Was this really just a disagreement about masks? Was it really just an individual objecting to a rule or a right-wing fanatic reacting to what she perceived as a left-wing policy? In energetic terms it was more than that.

As the new consciousness rises and many of us experience our blinders slipping off, giving us intimations of a larger perspective, there is at the same time a reactive intensification of "us versus them" thinking. There's a generalized rise in fractiousness, showing up in people's behaviors in public and online.

And it's not a matter of enlightened people staying calm while ignorant old-school thinkers become inflamed. Most of us have experienced reactivity no matter where we sit on the political spectrum. Most of us have found ourselves getting triggered, feeling outrage, and sometimes involuntarily striking out or shutting down.

This is because the mechanism that keeps you in your body, focused in the here and now — your *gatekeeper* — does not like change!

Your gatekeeper is a feature built into all your energy systems that keeps the gates of self. It says: "This is me; this is not me," "This is safe; this is not safe," "This belongs; this needs to be repelled," "This is friend; this is invader." It serves a very crucial role in keeping you, as a soul/spirit choosing to have a human experience, in your body.

On the *physical level,* your gatekeeper is your immune system. It determines what is accepted or rejected in your body. When you have inflammation, allergic reactions, aches and pains, physical accidents, and other symptoms, that is your gatekeeper giving warnings about your body's functioning or needs. Your gatekeeper is also the mechanism that funds energy for healing processes when it perceives healing as the safest and best choice.

On the *energetic level,* it is your boundary keeper and bouncer. It triages which energies can enter your field and which must be repelled, sometimes with quite strong force. It can influence how your subtle energies move and behave in its mission to keep you safe and sound.

On the *emotional level,* it animates feelings of attraction and aversion, guiding you toward and away from various people and experiences. It provides a flood of emotions, meant to give you information about the choices you make. When you meet someone and have an instant sense of discomfort, that is your gatekeeper signaling you to pay attention and assess the situation.

On the *mental level,* it activates involuntary thoughts and is that voice in your head offering a carrot and a stick: tempting, cajoling, criticizing, warning, and framing the experience in line with earlier lived experience. If triggered, it can come up with a total misinterpretation that you are certain is the truth, flattening your perceptions to black/white thinking.

On the *spiritual level,* your gatekeeper is a conduit for inner guidance, fueling certain projects and shutting down others, sometimes influencing the course of events in quite startling ways. But also, when your gatekeeper is triggered into reactivity, it can make it extremely difficult to hear inner guidance without distortion and can create an unholy mess.

On the *collective level,* groups of people have a shared gatekeeper protecting the web of connections they have established. This group gatekeeper often moves energetically to attract and repel individual souls and to referee membership in the group. It is usually reflected in the rules and beliefs people carry about who belongs and who doesn't, who is acceptable and who must be denied.

The gatekeeper is not a metaphor! It is part of how your body and mind are structured energetically to provide an instrument for your spirit to experience this earth dimension.

My Councils ascribe four major tasks to this mechanism:

1. **Keeping you safe and sound.** The gatekeeper maintains your boundaries and definition.
2. **Building and protecting your identity.** It keeps the map of self that guides how you navigate and create experiences.
3. **Maintaining habits.** It is the manager of your autopilot. Although your conscious choices help to set up the habits, once your gatekeeper has stored them, your body will respond according to the script and replay an experience, unless you consciously overwrite it.
4. **Allocating energies.** On the basis of your stored identity and habits, your gatekeeper energetically funds some things and defunds others. Its first funding priority uses "protect you" as its criteria. Second priority, it funds to maintain the sanctity and identity of your three selves (Earth Elemental Self, Talking Self, and Wiser Self). Third priority, it provides you with information about issues with your inner and outer functioning.

The fractiousness, reactivity, and even the black/white thinking we are seeing in people who were not previously so polarized are all symptoms of a triggered gatekeeper, signaling that the self feels violated or unsafe.

It is important to know this: the heightened discord we are seeing is not emanating from the topic, political stance, belief, or rules themselves.

These may be gatekeeper *triggers*, but gatekeeper *reactivity* is an energetic phenomenon that we all experience and that we can address and work with!

BEFRIENDING YOUR GATEKEEPER

As a young man, Stan felt strong spiritual stirrings. After reading a combination of Catholic and Buddhist teachings, he decided to embrace the notion of "no self." He gave away all his worldly possessions and launched himself onto the mercy of the world at large, wandering as a modern-day pilgrim.

Unfortunately, he did not take into account his own gatekeeper needs. Within weeks he developed anemia, he lost mental focus, and his wandering became a dazed meander rather than an ecstatic connection with spirit in the world.

Furthermore, forgetting his inter-connectedness with friends and acquaintances (and their gatekeepers), he triggered a panicked outcry from friends who read his farewell note — "I am done with all this worldly nonsense" — as a suicide declaration and contacted the FBI to track him down.

When they caught up with him, he was hospitalized for two weeks to stabilize his blood and then sent home to his parents, who enlisted their local priest to help guide Stan's spiritual quest with some more structured teachings.

His gatekeeper had refused to fund the project of no self he craved. And it had sounded the alarm physically, mentally, and socially.

As we awaken spiritually and our awareness of having a self shifts to a more global, we-are-one focus, it is tempting to try to jettison the self and the gatekeeper with it. But most of the people I have worked with who attempted this got strong blowback from their bodies or minds. I suspect that as long as you are in a body, you will need a gatekeeper to keep this body functioning as a unit.

Can you imagine if every time you came in range of another human being or creature, your own body rhythms just merged with and took on the functioning of that other being? Like an energy chameleon, your heart would shift its beat, your body would experience the illnesses and identity of the other, and you would be plunged into whatever thoughts and negativity and pain the other was carrying.

If you say yes, you have experienced this, then you are a highly sensitive empath, and this chapter is especially relevant for you. Your gatekeeper needs to learn better skills to distinguish the "me" from the "not me" in order for your body and life story not to involuntarily just mush into all that is.

Does this mean you are stuck with this limiting binary mechanism that sometimes seems to rule your body and mind? Not at all. Having a working gatekeeper does not impair your ability to feel compassion, open your consciousness, or become enlightened. The goal — and now it is becoming an imperative — is to befriend and partner with your gatekeeper and help it evolve toward spherical consciousness. Fortunately, there is lots of energy medicine and lifestyle medicine you can use to accomplish this.

UNDERSTANDING REACTIVITY

Psychologists and physicians talk about the fight, flight, or freeze reactions as part of our autonomic nervous system. *Autonomic* is, in my mind, a fancy term for the gatekeeper autopilot feature.

But it is useful to dive a bit deeper into reactivity, since most of us experience a glorious rainbow of reactions that we don't always recognize as our gatekeeper getting triggered.

For one thing, it is useful to know that you have a *yang gatekeeper* protecting you from threats to your identity in the world, body, and physical self. And you have a *yin gatekeeper* that protects the inner sense of self and the inner sanctity of your self.

Fight and flight are reactions of the yang gatekeeper, preparing to vanquish or get you physically out of the situation.

Freeze tends to be more a function of your yin gatekeeper, protecting you from hurt or invasion.

I generally add in other reactions, such as *fog*, which is what the squid does when it squirts ink in the water to obscure it from view. In people, fogging can take the form of putting out vibes that leave people around you befuddled and scrambled, or it can take the form of lots of inconsequential chatter that causes people to stop attending to you.

⚭ Play with It! ⚭

What form of reactivity does your gatekeeper use to protect your body and mind from invaders or to protect your inner sanctity of self? Try this "Gatekeeper Reactivity Self-Assessment" to see how your gatekeeper likes to roll. This is not an exhaustive or scientific assessment — just a chance to explore the creative ways your gatekeeper expresses itself!

Gatekeeper Reactivity Self-Assessment

Rate on a scale of 0 to 10 how often during a week you are in this state of reactivity:

0 = never, 3 = occasionally, 5 = once a day, 7 = a few times a day, 9 or 10 = several times a day.

(Note: if you score 5 or above for most items, you can adjust the scale to assess how many times *each day* you experience each of these.)

How often does your yang gatekeeper react with:

Fight (react, argue, strike out, get prickly, try to control a conversation, obstruct): _____

Flight (leave, hang up, ghost people, change the subject, stop trying, distract, procrastinate): _____

Flood (talk fast, run adrenaline, overeat or engage in other addictive behaviors, multitask): _____

Flutter (dodge the ball by jumping here and there, being all over the place, being unable to focus or concentrate, exhibiting ADHD): _____

Fiddle (rationalize, pick holes in or criticize, box with something, nitpick, get obsessed with minutiae or OCD kinds of tasks): _____

Tally your responses above and divide by 5 to get your yang gate-keeper reactivity estimate: _____

How often does your yin gatekeeper react with:

Freeze (like a deer in headlights; also can take the form of physical blockage or congestion): _____

Fog (obscure or confuse, like a squid squirts ink or skunk makes stink): _____

Fade (get vague, disappear, go into denial, get drained): _____

Fatigue (no energy, too tired or achy to function): _____

Faint (literal fainting, brownout of body functions, vasovagal reactions): _____

Fall apart (act helpless, come unglued, overemote or emote all over the place, become a puddle): _____

Fumble (get clumsy, stutter, become unable to form sentences or grasp things): _____

Falter (have surges and crashes, skip beats, hesitate, knock your rhythm off, create arrhythmia, show inability to stay on task): _____

Fail (shutdown of organs, mind, heart, gut; stopping any forward motion; mental, emotional, or physical paralysis): _____

Fibrillate (heartbeat or breath go into overdrive or dysregulation): _____

Tally your yin gatekeeper scores and divide by 10 to get your yin gatekeeper reactivity estimate: _____

⚭ • ⚭

All the *f*'s of reactivity are energetic reactions that affect your body's chemistry, your muscular-skeletal balance, your nervous system, your ability to break down and process toxins, and your capacity to build up new, healthy cells. They influence your mind and emotions. Consider what happens when you *freeze* in an important interview or *flood* your body with too much data during a difficult time in your life. These reactions impact you on all the levels at which the gatekeeper is protecting you, often blocking your comfort and access to your inner guidance system.

Therefore, once you realize that you are experiencing your gatekeeper in action, it is important to learn to:

1. calm the reactivity
2. clean up the mess left in its wake (by rebalancing your energies)
3. address what your gatekeeper has communicated about your needs for safety, authentic identity, self-supportive habits, and better pathways of energy distribution

The gatekeeper is your agent, meant to facilitate your creation of self, not your jailer, bent on keeping you in a prison of reactivity, restriction, and dysfunction.

CALM GATEKEEPER REACTIVITY

Donna Eden, whose teachings have awakened many to their larger energetic nature, tells a wonderful story about calming the gatekeeper, which she calls the Triple Warmer.

She was strolling down a street one day in Sausalito, California, enjoying some sunshine. Ahead of her, she noticed a disturbance. She saw people startling, turning, and barreling away from the sidewalk, and she heard shouting but couldn't distinguish the words.

She kept walking toward the disturbance, until she could see the problem: a rabid dog was raging its way toward her, foaming at the mouth and baring its teeth. Her immediate instinct was to engage the dog's energies.

Although the dog was about forty feet away, she reached out with her hands and energetically made contact with that poor dog's Triple Warmer, calming it with motions I describe below in the exercise "Pet the Doggy / Pet the Kitty." As she soothed that dog's Triple Warmer meridian — the energy stream most linked with yang reactivity — she first saw the dog stop in its tracks. Then it looked around, as if confused. Then it dropped down on its belly, as if pinned in place. And it stayed there as Donna continued to sedate its Triple Warmer until animal rescue arrived.

It is extremely useful to have a whole pocketful of simple techniques for calming the gatekeeper in a moment of reactivity and to practice them on yourself whenever you find your gatekeeper has gotten triggered. (However, if a rabid dog is running toward you, running away is still an excellent first-choice strategy.)

Normally, it is your own gatekeeper you need to release from reactivity, but most of the techniques I offer below will work on others (with their permission) when you are able to truly enter the energy stream or interact with the energy field in question. Donna Eden had fortunately developed that skill in healing herself and supporting others. And you can too.

A POCKETFUL OF SIMPLE ENERGY TECHNIQUES TO CALM THE GATEKEEPER

Exercise: Pet the Doggy / Pet the Kitty

I use this exercise to quickly pull my gatekeeper out of reactivity or to help clients who need to respond to their gatekeepers but don't necessarily want to learn a lot of complicated energy medicine. (Note: this is a variation on a Donna Eden exercise called the "Triple Warmer Smoothie.") Here's how to do it for yourself:

1. Ask yourself, "Which do you prefer, dogs or cats?" Choosing a pet you relate to helps to activate the soothing, loving energies in your hands.
2. Place one hand on each temple, beside your eyes. Starting there, pet the doggy or kitty by stroking with all your fingertips up over the ears, down behind the ears, and down the sides of the neck, letting your hands rest, with comforting solidity, on the collarbone by the base of your neck. It can enhance the calming energy to croon, "good doggy" or "good kitty" while you stroke.
3. Cross your arms so your right hand is on your left collarbone and your left hand is on your right collarbone. Then continue petting down both arms at once, your right hand stroking the

back of your left arm and your left hand stroking the back of your right arm.

This stroking motion travels against the flow along the pathway of what I call your *energizer stream* (called Triple Warmer meridian in Chinese medicine; see figure 6.2, page 131). By stroking against the flow, you calm it.

4. Repeat this petting motion slowly and lovingly, bringing all the love you feel for your dog or cat to your own body, until you can feel your gatekeeper settling down and relaxing.

5. To end the exercise, place both hands over your heart for the duration of at least three deep breaths.

∞ • ∞

In the midst of a crisis, when your gatekeeper is reacting and you need to calm it quickly, having an exercise like "Pet the Doggy / Pet the Kitty" in your repertoire is excellent.

I use many different methods to calm my gatekeeper, depending on the circumstances. My two favorites act to reset major circuit breakers. My go-to for resetting the yang gatekeeper is "Porcupine Reset." (If you've taken my classes or read *The Language Your Body Speaks*, you already know "Porcupine Reset," because I think it is a crucial bit of energy dialogue and I included it in that book.) For releasing a frozen yin gatekeeper, I generally start with "Flip Your Halos" (see page 104).

Protocol: Porcupine Reset

This exercise resets your body's polarities. When your yang gatekeeper goes into reactivity, it will start flipping polarities in your energy field, like energy switches directing your body's energies where to go and what to do. You will probably feel prickly like a porcupine, frantic, angry, nettled, scared, or frazzled. "Porcupine Reset" helps flip the master switch, getting your energies back into correct orientation. This will often stop overall electromagnetic reactivity. Repeat the sequence as many times as needed to break the reactivity.

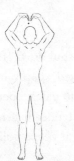

1. Starting at the top of the head, grab the energy with two hands.

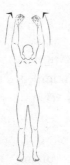

2. On the inhale, pull it straight up to arm's length.

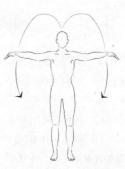

3. On the exhale, pull it down on either side of your body, arcing out in an egg-shaped arc.

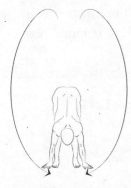

4. Tack the energy to the floor.

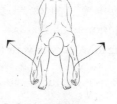

5. Grab energy from the earth.

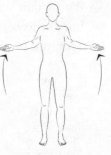

6. On the inhale, pull it up with both hands, arcing out.

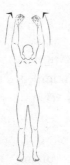

7. On the exhale, tack it to the top of the head.

Figure 5.1. Porcupine Reset

Protocol: Flip Your Halos

When your yin gatekeeper gets triggered, you may feel shut down, unable to process, faint, emotionally swamped, discombobulated, spacey, listless, lacking in purpose, or clueless. That's because your yin gatekeeper protects the inner sanctity of your self — your beautiful tender heart, your soul's truth, your deepest values, your inner knowing. It keeps pollution out, but sometimes it also locks you in.

To calm this reactivity:

1. First, draw the longitudinal lines of a sphere around you, using your hands to create it as described in "Anchoring in the Stabilizing Sphere" (pages 88–92). This reminds your body of its orientation to all that is.

2. Then you are going to work with your four halos (see figure 5.2):

    •   The *main halo* is eight inches above your head.

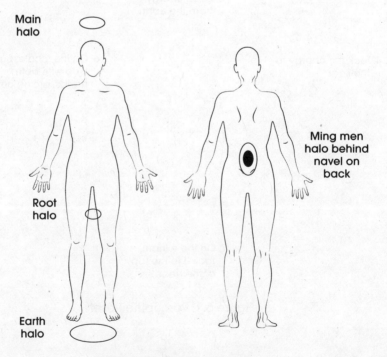

Figure 5.2. Your four halos

- Your *root halo* is eight inches below your groin.
- Your *earth halo* is eight inches below your feet.
- Your *ming men halo* is on your body (not eight inches away) at your ming men area. This is directly behind your belly button, around the L2, L3, and L4 vertebrae, between your kidneys.

3. Starting with your main halo, grasp it on both sides, the way you would grasp a Frisbee. Inhale. Then flip it as you exhale, so the upper side now faces down. Feel into it. If it felt better the other way around, flip it back. If it feels better with this new orientation, leave it.

4. Now grasp your root halo on both sides, the way you would grasp a Frisbee. Inhale. Flip it as you exhale, so the bottom becomes the top. Feel into it. Does this feel better or worse? If it is better, leave it; if it is worse, flip it back.

5. Then, if you are able, sit with your knees bent and feet pulled toward you (see figure 5.3), so you can reach your earth halo, eight inches below your feet. If this position doesn't work for you, imagine your arms are loooong and reach down as if to grasp both sides of the halo.

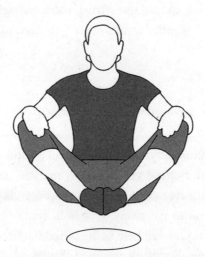

Figure 5.3. Body position to reach your earth halo

Inhale. Flip the halo as you exhale, so the side that was facing you now faces away. Does this feel better or worse? If it is better, leave it. If you feel worse, flip it back.

6.   Reach behind your back to your ming men halo. Grasp it with one or both hands (depending on your flexibility). Inhale. Then flip it as you exhale, so the side that faced your body now faces away. Feel into it. If it is better, leave it. If it is worse, flip it back.

Note: you can adjust any of these to work better for you physically, using a combination of gesture and intention. My friend who can't reach behind her back first leans against a cushion to activate her ming men halo, then adjusts it out in front of her, sending the message to her back. Energy is not as dense as physical matter and can move beautifully with a combination of touch, gesture, and intention!

The four halos, being electromagnetic circuit breakers, will toggle open and closed. The reason I invite you to feel into each one is to determine whether you have opened a closed circuit (as you intended) or closed an open one.

If you know how to energy test (see appendix A), you can test each halo by *energy localizing*— placing your hand on each halo — and testing. Palm facing the body should test strong; palm facing away from the body should test weak. Any other results mean you need to flip the halo.

∽ • ∾

Here are some additional simple strategies to calm your gatekeeper:

- **Put one hand on your forehead and another on the back of your head, behind your eyes.** When you go into reactivity, the blood leaves your forebrain and travels into the legs to prepare you to run away. This hold (an Eden Energy Medicine technique) will help bring blood back to your forebrain, so you can make more reasoned choices.

- **Submerse yourself in water (shower, bath, a jump in the** lake) or cover your face with a wet washcloth. Water calms the fire of reactivity. Although any energy system can act on behalf of the gatekeeper, there is a central office for this mechanism in the element of fire and in your energy streams that represent fire.

- **Practice three-five breathing: breathe in on a count of three and out on a count of five, making your exhale longer than your inhale.** The yin gatekeeper often causes breath to freeze or falter, and the yang gatekeeper often causes you to breathe faster or more raggedly. Three-five breathing helps to reset your in-out rhythm and to release the overenergized expressions of your reactivity. It also calms your vagus nerve, which is part of your yin gatekeeper communication system.

- **Hold hands with the Divine: literally use your hand to grasp something you associate with the Divine or act out holding hands with the Divine.** Your gatekeeper's cosmic partner is radiance, your soul, your animating force. When you hold hands with the Divine, you bring in this partner to remind the gatekeeper that in your essence, you are safe, bigger than your specific story lines, and able to make conscious choices.

- **Lie flat on the earth and entrain to her, letting the earth breathe you.** This practice is not recommended for the grocery store! If it isn't possible for you to lie on the earth, grasping a round stone or bouncing a ball can help. Dropping into entrainment with an integrated spherical consciousness will often release the binary reactivity of the gatekeeper.

- **Cross your arms or interlace your fingers and breathe slowly in and out.** As in "Open Sesame" (below), this action integrates your left and right brains and brings you into the circle consciousness of your breath. Interlacing your fingers helps your energy streams to work together more effectively, calming a gatekeeper that feels unsupported and at risk.

- **Count to ten or engage in any other simple number medicine, like counting by twos or threes.** This can rapidly bring structure to your energies and focus your mind, which often

gets bombarded with spiraling "stinking thinking" when the
gatekeeper is triggered.

- **Hug a tree or bring your body into contact with some other
  structure (a wall, a box) and allow it to "console" your gatekeeper.** Hugging a tree brings your three densities (Earth
  Elemental Self, Talking Self, and Wiser Self) into alignment
  and brings perspective to the part of you in reactivity. Holding or leaning on a structure lends your energies structure.

Protocol: Open Sesame

For use when you are experiencing resistance, fear, or jumping out of your
skin. Also helpful if you are feeling fragmented or shattered or disconnected in some way. This simple protocol tells your body, mind, and spirit
that you are showing up for yourself, and it brings integration and unity
to energies that are chaotic or disjunct.

1. Take your gatekeeper out of porcupine reactivity by doing the
   "Porcupine Reset" (pages 102–3).
2. Interlace the fingers of both hands and put them over your
   heart, until you feel your heart is calm and centered (see figure 5.4).

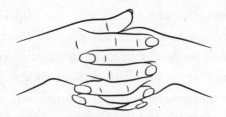

Figure 5.4. Interlaced fingers

3. Then place your interlaced hands over your forehead, until
   you feel your thoughts or mind calming.
4. Now, place your interlaced fingers on the back of your head,

behind your eyes, and hold there until you feel a measure of release from fear. (If you wish, you can vary the order of steps 2, 3, and 4.)

5. Then, if you can reach, interlace your fingers at the ming men area of your back (behind your belly button, around the L2, L3, and L4 vertebrae, between your kidneys) and hold until you feel yourself opening to deeper truths.

    If you can't reach your back, do this hold in front of your second chakra, between the belly button and pubic bone, until you feel you are in touch with your authentic self.

6. Finally, *don the robes of your larger service* (whatever larger purpose you serve), using gestures or a scarf or an actual robe or uniform to evoke the feeling of donning your robes. Feel the robes settle and allow yourself to be that role. If you do not know what larger purpose you serve, just don the robes of service to the earth or whatever cause you would like to dedicate your day to.

If you can't physically do these holds, here are some alternative options:

•   Using one hand, hold something woven or an image of a Celtic knot at each of the positions listed above. (The version of the Celtic knot in figure 5.5, with interspersed hearts, is especially potent.)

•   If your tension arises from being cut off from nature, you can use a green leaf picked from a tree or plant (ask permission

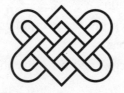

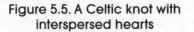

Figure 5.5. A Celtic knot with
interspersed hearts

of the plant!) at each of the positions, with or without the hands interlaced. That will integrate your energies with nature again.

∞ • ∞

CLEAN UP THE MESS

After a storm, there is usually a mess to clean up: your yard is littered with leaves and branches and garbage that has blown in, your roof or windows need to be repaired, and the lawn furniture has to be put back in order. Downed trees need clearing, and any downed electric lines have to be reinstated. If the storm was a hurricane, you'll remove storm shutters and clean up from flooding. If it was a tornado, you may be looking at a major rebuild or community-wide cleanup campaign.

This is pretty much the situation in your body when your gatekeeper gets triggered and communicates its reactivity in myriad ways:

- It floods your body with stress hormones.
- It tightens and sometimes torques muscles (or releases them so they are too loose).
- It causes the subtle energies that run your body to flow irregularly (backward or in odd rhythms or at too-high and too-low levels).

It can, among other things:

- Shut down digestion
- Instruct cells to reproduce too rapidly
- Stop healing processes
- Convert reproductive and digestive hormones to stress hormones
- Cause your brain to go blank or go into overdrive
- Set loose feelings, ungrounded thoughts, and frantic behaviors, knocking your sense of time and place askew

Your gatekeeper will do whatever it feels is necessary to keep you alive, including threaten the very life it is designed to preserve! Autoimmune reactions are superstrong gatekeeper communications, telling you there is a serious problem with your safety, identity, habits, or energy usage or with your relationship with being in a body and with gatekeeping itself.

Although any energy system of your body can act as a gatekeeper, certain physical and energy systems are involved most often in gatekeeper reactivity:

- Your nervous system — the body's electrics
- Your grounding — the energetic polarities, the flow of energies in your aura or energy field
- Your blood chemistry and immune system responses
- Your meridians, which are energy streams that (among other things) fuel the work of the body and your organs
- Your hormones and the glands that regulate them, including the adrenals, thyroid, hypothalamus, pituitary, and pineal
- Your organs that help produce and process messaging hormones, including your liver, large and small intestines, heart, stomach, gallbladder, and spleen
- Your microbiome — the microorganisms that help to regulate your health
- Your brain, which reacts to electrical dysregulation in the body

Too much information? This isn't an invitation to start chasing monkeys. The good news is that *anything* you do to befriend your gatekeeper will act as a banana to reinstate healthy balance and flow. And as you proceed in this book — learning tools for grounding, centering, rooting, anchoring, reinstating coherence, supporting flow, reweaving your web of connections, and reconnecting with radiance — your gatekeeper will heal and evolve.

In the construction of your self, your gatekeeper truly does keep the gates of your existence and is central to any healing or evolution you wish to bring in. But by showing up, bringing your conscious attention, and perhaps adding some radiance, joy, love, or other illumination to the conversation, you will find your gatekeeper *wants* to work in partnership with you.

To simplify all of this, though, try the following exercises. To reset the communication pathways of your yang gatekeeper, do "Energy Relay Reset" (pages 114–16). To reset your yin gatekeeper, you can use "Gatekeeper Syncing" (pages 116–17). Sometimes these protocols will initiate spontaneous cleanup and save you a lot of work!

SUPPORT FOR YOUR YANG AND YIN

You are probably somewhat familiar with the sympathetic and parasympathetic nervous systems.

The sympathetic nervous system often deals with the fight-or-flight response. Sound familiar? Your yang gatekeeper uses your sympathetic nervous system to facilitate communication in your body.

The yang gatekeeper communicates via the four burners (see figure 5.6).

The yang gatekeeper uses a relay that includes the "organ" Chinese medicine refers to as the Triple Warmer (comprising the *dan tien* burner, solar plexus burner, and heart burner). It also includes the adrenal glands, the thyroid, and the hypothalamus, which is a master gland in your brain.

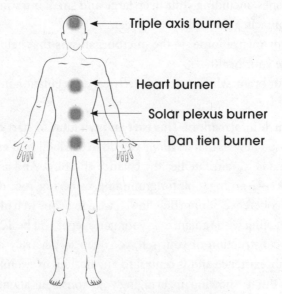

Figure 5.6. Your four burners

I call this fourth burner the *triple axis burner* because it sits in the area of your hypothalamus, pineal, and pituitary glands.

See "Energy Relay Reset" (pages 114–16) for a process to reinstate your yang gatekeeper circuit.

The parasympathetic nervous system initiates what is sometimes called the "rest and digest" or "breed and feed" responses. (What is it about reactivity that invites rhyming and alliteration?) Your yin gatekeeper uses your parasympathetic nervous system, and in particular your vagus nerve, to communicate in the body.

Your yin gatekeeper communicates via the vagus nerve, heart, and circulatory system (see figure 5.7).

The vagus is a wandering nerve that touches most of your organs and serves as a communication superhighway for yin gatekeeping.

See "Gatekeeper Syncing" on pages 116–17 for a process to reinstate your yin gatekeeper communications.

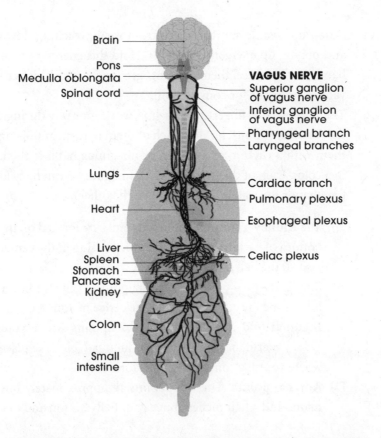

Figure 5.7. The vagus nerve touches most of your organs

Protocol: Energy Relay Reset

This is an excellent exercise for cleaning up after a yang gatekeeper storm. It is also great if you are experiencing adrenal fatigue, thyroid issues, or other energy distribution challenges.

Don't be intimidated by all the points in the diagram below. Your body has all kinds of *energy access points* that allow you to connect to and communicate with your subtle energies. You do not need to know energy anatomy to use them. You can follow the instructions below as a kind of paint-by-numbers experience.

However, as you are holding each point or set of points, pay attention. Listen. See what it feels like to be holding that particular place on your body. The more you treat this as a getting-acquainted activity and as an exercise in showing up for yourself, the more you will get out of it.

1. Scoop up cosmic source energy from earth, reaching down and pulling up energetic nutrients. Hold this energy in your hands until you feel them opening, growing warm. This activates your hands for conversation.

2. Then, using your fingertips or palms, work your way through the following points, holding each of them in turn, or pulsing them with a rhythm or a sound, or imagining bathing them in a color. Each of the pairs of points in figure 5.8 can be held together or separately (one side, then the other):

   A) **The Kidney-1 points.** These acupoints are located on the bottom of each foot, in the slight depression at the center next to the ball of the foot.

   B) **The Kidney-10 points.** These acupoints points sit in the fold of the knee, on the inside back edge of your leg.

   C) **Inguinal fold points.** These are acupoints where your kidney meridian flow crosses the inguinal fold (the place where your leg connects to your torso).

   D) **Adrenal points.** These acupoints sit approximately one to one and a half inches above your belly button and one

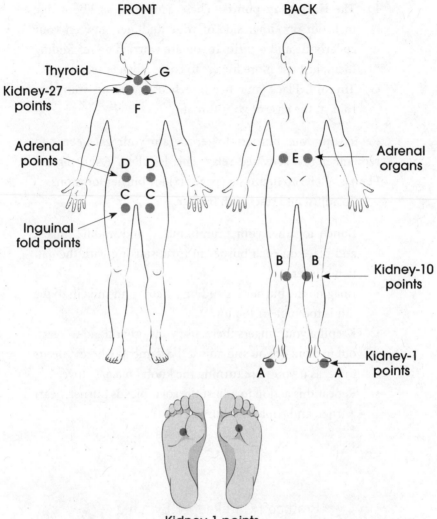

FRONT

BACK

Thyroid

G

Kidney-27 points

F

Adrenal points

D   D

C   C

Inguinal fold points

Adrenal organs

E

B   B

Kidney-10 points

Kidney-1 points

A   A

Kidney-1 points

Figure 5.8. Energy relay reset points

to one and a half inches to either side. If you press in on these points, they are generally sore if they need support.

E) **Adrenal organs on the back.** Place your hands on your sides at your waist. Slide your fingers around to cover your lower back, where your kidney and adrenal glands sit.

F) **The Kidney-27 points.** These acupoints sit about one inch out on either side of your midline, between your collarbone and top rib. If you are worried about finding them, just use more fingers to cover a bigger territory.

G) **Thyroid.** Place your five bunched fingers on your thyroid, at the base of your throat.

3. Reset your four burners to reprogram your gatekeeper to remember this activated relay. This is called "Adjusting the Flames." Refer to figure 5.6 (page 112) for burner locations.

   To adjust and reset each burner:

   • Bunch together your thumb, index, and middle fingers and place on each burner in turn, starting with the dan tien burner.

   • Imagine the burner is exuding a flame and tune in to see if it is too high or too low.

   • Keeping your fingers there, use your other hand to reach out in front of you and adjust the flame to where it needs to be, as if you were turning the knob on a gas stove.

   • Repeat this action to adjust the solar plexus burner, heart burner, and triple axis burner.

☯ • ☯

Protocol: Gatekeeper Syncing

This exercise is great for cleaning up and resetting yin communications after your yin gatekeeper has shut down or reacted.

1. Place one hand flat on your heart (as if doing the Pledge of Allegiance). With your other hand, hold hands with the Divine, as explained on page 107. (I usually grasp with my actual hand while picturing or feeling the Goddess holding my hand.) Do this until you feel calm and connected with the Divine. If you

don't believe in a Divine, hold hands with whatever you feel most dedicated to: truth, beauty, peace.

2. Place one hand along the side of your neck (on either side) to key into your vagus nerve. While holding that, hook up the side of your neck with your heart by placing your other palm flat on your heart.

3. Keeping one hand along the side of your neck, use your other hand to connect in with each of the four burners. If you desire, you can include "Clearing Templates from the Temples" (pages 125–26) while doing this hold and invite the Universal Supply Team to help you carry out any needed cleanup work.

4. Now, still with a hand on the side of your neck over the vagus nerve, use your other hand to connect your vagus nerve up with any other places on your body, such as organs or meridians, that you instinctively feel need yin connection. (Once you have learned to enter the stream in chapter 6, try this with your heart/connection stream or choice/discernment stream in particular.)

5. End by holding one hand on your heart while holding hands with the Divine with your other hand.

�∞ • ∞

In the next chapter, "Enter the Stream," we will explore the third aspect of partnering with your gatekeeper: how to deepen your relationship with your subtle energies and evolve your gatekeeper beyond binary consciousness.

∽ Chapter Six ∽

Enter the Stream

Did you ever notice that most disembodied guides tend to be male? Seth, Bartholomew, Abraham...I have loved their teachings, but always wondered, *Where are the wise dead women?* And when people talk about their spirit guides, why do they always seem to be Native Americans or East Indians? Were there no wise Iowa farmers sticking around to guide us in our earthbound journeys? You just don't hear about someone getting cosmic messages from Maude or Homer!

My young feminist self was relieved (and secretly feeling a bit superior) when my inner teachers turned out to be group consciousnesses, without marked gender or national identities. When I asked them about their nature, my Councils explained that all channeled material is shaped by the instrument that receives it, even if that person is apparently not conscious of the transmissions. My mind, they said, would naturally receive their energy as collective, nongendered, and multicultural.

You can imagine my surprise, then, the day the Old Chinese Gentleman showed up in my practice room to guide me in helping a client. It was in the first year of my accidental new healing career, when people were just hearing about me via word of mouth and calling to ask for sessions.

I borrowed a massage table and agreed to see people if they would also work with a licensed practitioner as a backup.

My client was lying facedown on the table, and I was idly watching my hands move over her body, just listening and noticing what I was feeling, letting my hands talk and my instincts take the lead. Suddenly I heard a voice say, "Hold out your hand." I looked up and saw an Old Chinese Gentleman standing near the table. A stereotypical Old Chinese Gentleman spirit of ancient mien, with a long, thin beard and a long gown. He nodded as if to say hello or maybe, "Hop to it."

I held out my hand. He placed a thin (energetic) gold needle on my palm and indicated with his eyes, *Insert it there.* His gaze traveled to my client's back, and the spot he was looking at just seemed to light up. *OK,* I thought, *why not?* I had never received acupuncture, but I once watched someone getting it. So I gently inserted the energetic gold needle where he indicated, miming the action as if it were an actual needle. He then handed me a silver needle and indicated with a nod a second point that was now lit up on her back. I gently eased the silver needle into place.

"Set it for fifteen minutes." He had so far not spoken much at all. I wondered, *Is it OK to ask, "Why set a timer?"* His face was not so much forbidding as decorous, serene. It felt gauche to inquire, "What are we doing?" So I rubbed the silver needle between my fingers and set the intention that it would dissolve in fifteen minutes. He nodded. I thought, *Now what?*

Suddenly, my client spoke up: "Are you doing acupuncture back there?"

"Why do you ask?"

"Because," she said, "it feels just like getting acupuncture."

That was the beginning of my adventures with "ghost acupuncture," as I dubbed it, just one more weirdo phenomenon in my increasingly woo-woo existence.

The Old Chinese Gentleman was a teacher of few words. Somehow the direction he gave me would just translate into a knowing in my head or body. I sometimes wondered if he even spoke English, because when I *heard* him, it was with my whole being, not merely sounds in my ears or head.

He showed up often for a few months, guiding me where to put the gold needle to act as the polestar and the silver needle to tonify or create movement. Eventually he had me add in platinum needles to deepen the healing work and copper needles for grounding. And before you ask, no, I have no idea if platinum was known in ancient China.

What I have learned about the Old Chinese Gentleman since was that he had many lifetimes as a healer spanning many cultures and times. In the particular lifetime from which he appeared to me, he practiced an ancient form of Chinese shamanism and was involved in the early creation of Chinese five-element healing and acupuncture.

Once he got the ball rolling, I found that even when he wasn't apparent in my practice room, I would notice places lighting up on my clients' bodies and just know where to put the polestar and tonifiers, the deepeners and grounding needles. And my clients' energies would shift, balance, resolve, and heal.

Then one day, as I got ready to place a gold energy needle in a spot that lit up on my client's back, I saw the Old Chinese Gentleman out of the corner of my eye and heard the words "Enter the stream." I signaled back with my eyes: "What?!" He nodded and showed me, with his gaze, the path of the energy stream where the acupoint was lit up. *Enter the stream.*

Tracing the line of the stream that was lit up on her back, I found a spot where I felt a pull. I shut my eyes and just dropped down into the energies, and all my senses expanded as I looked around me and felt my way into the movement and sensations of the landscape I found myself in. I heard words and sounds; I smelled woody smells (and later discovered it was a meridian pathway associated with wood element). It was the first and maybe only time when I dropped into an energy stream and *all* my senses activated at once. Like a kid in a candy store, I did not need to be guided to explore: the stream just called to me, and I wandered and marveled.

After a while, the place began to speak to me of what it needed. I noticed things in this inner landscape I was experiencing: a place where the water was clogged by a tree that had fallen over; an area where someone had planted stakes, as if to build a fence, and left them there to rot. And I called on the Universal Supply Team to help me do what I could to address those needs.

When I had completed the work, emerged out of the stream, and finished the healing session, my client reported feeling a profound shift. Over the next few months, we learned just how profound: the cancer we had been trying to address went into remission and then cleared out of her system.

That moment was a major turning point for me in my evolution as a healer and as a person. It was the moment when I understood that energy work is not an outside-in activity. It is an inside job.

ADDRESS THE COMMUNICATION: DEEPER WORK WITH YOUR GATEKEEPER

Going inside is not something our culture emphasizes, and so for many of us, the first time we ask, inside-out healing does not just light up in our awareness, and our bodies don't just automatically show us the way.

I was lucky, because I had tour guides and because I had spent years listening inward for inspiration, material for stories, ideas to write about. And because my latent gifts of being a messenger got activated fairly early in life, my ability to recognize what I was hearing and perceiving with my other senses was already in working order by the time the Old Chinese Gentleman invited me to enter the stream.

That said, the skill did not just show up fully developed. I spent hours and hours exploring my own inner byways, sometimes illuminated by what I found, sometimes unclear about what was happening or needed. But I kept showing up. Whenever I had a problem with a relationship, or a health challenge, or even a societal problem I wanted to investigate, I would drop into an energy stream or some part of my energetic makeup and let it teach me.

I would also often meet up for conversations with my Councils in diverse inner landscapes (and in a place they called "the country of the mind") rather than speaking for them into my typewriter or computer. And in my work with clients, I shifted from just following my hands and moving energies to helping them learn to participate in their own healing from the inside out.

Over time, I learned to:

- drop in and perceive
- interact
- open to new perspectives and symbolic guidance
- bring support to where my energies lived

And that is the invitation to learning energy conversations in this book. Let your body be the doorway to deeper knowing and broader consciousness.

On pages 46–48 I introduced an initial Guided Visit: "Cradle and Clear an Organ Space." If you tried it, what parts worked for you and what parts didn't? Some people get tons of images and impressions and story lines; others perceive or feel next to nothing. That doesn't mean nothing happened. There is an art to teaching your mind (and gatekeeper) to accept unfamiliar, new experiences. I believe it can be helpful to scaffold on what you already know.

Try the same activity, "Cradle and Clear an Organ Space," again. But this time, when you set your intention to drop into your chosen organ, imagine you are dropping into a room you have known at some point. Or an imaginary room, if you prefer. Now explore: What is the furniture, how do you feel about its placement? What is missing from this room, or what is extra that doesn't belong? What needs to happen in order for you to restore or renovate this room to its potential glory?

This technique of renovating and caring for a space helps you give some form to perceiving energies, which can seem hard to get a handle on if you just try to perceive them with a blank-slate mind.

When you have done your best to calm your gatekeeper and reinstate your energy circuitry, as described in chapter 5, the third step is working to communicate more deeply with your gatekeeper, in ways that help it to evolve from binary yes/no reactivity toward spherical both/and acceptance of diversity and inter-connection. In order to do that, I invite you to learn to *clear templates from your temples* and enter the streams most intimately connected with your gatekeeper: your *fire element* streams.

KEEPING THE FLAMES AND CARING FOR THE TEMPLES

Your gatekeeper moderates the distribution of energies in your body, including heat, fuel for the organs, and hormone messaging to guide the work of the body. Its home base for this activity is what I call your *four chambers* (see figure 6.1):

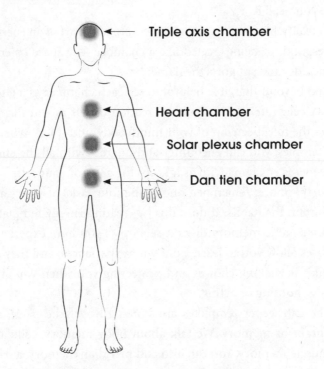

Triple axis chamber

Heart chamber

Solar plexus chamber

Dan tien chamber

Figure 6.1. Your four chambers

- The *dan tien chamber* is located at the second chakra, between the pubis and the belly button.
- The *solar plexus chamber* is located at the third chakra, at the solar plexus.
- The *heart chamber* is located in the center of the chest, next to your anatomical heart.
- The *triple axis chamber* is located at the sixth chakra, where the hypothalamus sits.

The exercise mentioned in chapter 5, "Adjusting the Flames" (page 116), works with the four burners or the flames that are energy feeds at the center of each chamber. Sometimes it is helpful to adjust the flames, the way you adjust the burners on your stove to get the proper level of heat under your pots. This will influence your hormones, your body's chemistry, your body's heating and cooling system, and your ability to distribute energy where you need it.

In reality, however, the four burners are each part of an energy complex that responds to being treated like a chamber — a space or environment that includes and supports the flame.

And beyond that, it is helpful to see each chamber as a temple where you can celebrate the miraculous creation of self as you form a life and express the full spectrum of your mind, body, and spirit. When you enter these temples, you can encounter and interact with all the energies your gatekeeper is engaging with as it keeps the gates of your self.

Furthermore, remember, one of the four tasks of your gatekeeper is to maintain the habits. It does this by creating energy templates — little coded energetic memory disks it sets up as you have experiences. These templates allow you to learn from your experiences, and they guide your autopilot in making choices and protecting you when you are not consciously choosing or acting.

The gatekeeper templates are stored all over the place, not just in your brain or memory. We talk about body memory, cellular memory, and muscle memory. You can also add meridian memory, auric memory, chakra memory, and chamber memory. Each of these is a fruitful place to enter the stream and explore what templates are guiding the ship.

If you are familiar with meridian tapping or EFT (Emotional Freedom Technique) tapping, you have already encountered a method of clearing gatekeeper templates. Through asking questions and bringing up topics, you call up the gatekeeper templates related to those issues. Then, as you tap specific acupoints, you are rebalancing your meridian energies, effectively telling your gatekeeper to stay balanced and energetically neutral in the face of that issue. You are overwriting the old templates with new instructions.

Tapping is great because it is simple and accessible and can make a profound difference. It works with your energy streams, which are major elements in your energetic makeup.

However, it doesn't always get at the templates of self stored in your chakras, your aura, and your temples. And it doesn't always allow you to write new templates in a holistic way. You might want to add the following template clearing to your repertoire.

As with all Guided Visits in this book, you can either record yourself reading it out loud, with pauses to allow yourself time to explore, or you can download an MP3 from ellenmeredith.com/visits, password: YBSW.

Guided Visit: Clearing Templates from the Temples

Find a place to lie down or sit comfortably, where you won't be interrupted. Place your hand flat over one of your chambers. (Use your intuition to choose one or just let your hand lead the way.) Take a moment to feel with your hand whatever sensations come up for you. Watch your breath come in and go out for at least three deep breaths and then sink your attention down into the chamber. It can help to imagine your inhale is opening the space for you and your exhale is carrying you down in.

Look for the flame. Where is it located? What does it need? You can adjust the flame by reaching out and imagining you are turning the knob on a gas stove, setting the flame to the level your hand instinctively feels it needs right now. Once you have reset the flame, trace a five-pointed star and circle on it to help it stay stable and to help the energies it represents stay balanced.

Now look, feel, sense around you to explore what this chamber is like. What is its shape, its decor, its ambiance? Where does the flame sit? Does it feel like a proper temple for the flame you just adjusted?

Who is here in the chamber with you? Do they belong, or do they perhaps need to be encouraged to move along?

Keep noticing what you can and ask your gatekeeper or the chamber itself to show you what you need to know about it. Let that dialogue take place in words, in symbols, in sensations, and in thoughts that enter your mind.

Remember you are getting to know the place. You don't have to fix things or interact extensively on this visit, unless you feel prepared to do so. Just dwell in the space and let it show you what it wants you to know. The flame is your own spirit, entering to fuel your gatekeeper's work of regulating your body and of funding your evolving self.

If you have things you feel block you from being well, write a sentence or two on a piece of (imaginary) paper, starting with, "My experience of ..." *My experience of overeating. My experience of self-insults. My experience with Peter.* And give that paper to the flame. You are not burning up Peter or decimating overeating for all time. It just helps to suggest to your gatekeeper to update its templates.

Now, if you want to plant seeds of a new behavior, belief, or way of walking in the world, do some symbolic action in the chamber to affirm that. You can call on positive teachers, make a wall mural or other piece of art, create an altar of gratitude, perform a short ritual, sing a song that expresses your new vision, or give yourself or the chamber a gift that symbolizes for you the change you'd like to invite in.

But be aware that the change should be an *essence* of what you want to cultivate, not a *form*.

If overeating is the problem, for example, you are not planting an image of yourself looking thin. Instead, plant a sense of yourself being comfortable with eating what your body needs in order to thrive. And if your relationship with Peter has been a problem, you're not planting a divorce decree; you are planting a seed of nourishing friendships and connections. The gatekeeper can understand essences you are asking it to call in. When you ask it to transform in specific ways, the request can backfire. You often just compound your gatekeeper's desire to bring you experiences that will allow you to grow beyond your attachment to those ways!

Who is the keeper of the flame, and who is the guardian of this temple? If you wish, you can call in a keeper or guardian to help protect and care for your flame.

When you are ready, thank them for their service and thank the space for your interactions today.

Bring your attention to your hand resting on your body and use your breath to lift yourself out of the chamber and back into awareness of your body sitting or lying down. Watch your inhales and exhales for three more deep breaths, and if you need to, gently pat yourself on your belly, arms, and legs to return to full presence in your body.

☙ • ☙

There is no rule about what to do when you travel into a space to interact with your energies where they live. Here is a list of some possible things you can do when you enter a stream or energetic space:

- Explore and discover; look around and see what is going on.
- Repair or renovate (with the help of the Universal Supply Team).
- Create a container to give the space better boundaries or repair the existing container.
- Balance energies using energy medicine exercises or symbolic actions.
- Dwell in a particular energy state or place you find there (for example, hang out in a garden or swim in a pool that shows up).
- Ask for guidance; seek visions.
- Conduct ritual work or spiritual practices (such as setting up an altar in the temple to support the flame).
- Encounter and interact with beings or work through scenes the way you'd do in active dreaming.
- Take a journey, follow pathways, go through doorways, and the like.
- Plant seeds of change.
- Make pacts with the guides or with yourself there, including rewriting contracts.

HOW DO YOU WANT TO INFLUENCE THE FLOW?

First listen, ask, learn. Explore the energies and use whatever language or perceptual understanding you have to characterize what you are experiencing.

Some questions to ask:

- Is the energy blocked or overly active?
- Is the place lacking or needing something?
- Is the place polluted or filled with the wrong contents in some

way? Or perhaps you've found yourself in the wrong landscape altogether?

- Is the energy or place you find yourself in too condensed or crowded — or, conversely, too dispersed or sparse?
- Is the energy you are exploring continuous and flowing, or does it feel disconnected or obstructed?
- Is the energy following a wrong path or needing a course correction?
- Is the stream or space overly full or underfilled?
- Who is there with you?
- What are the strengths of this stream or place that you can build on?

Whenever I teach entering the streams, I inevitably find a few people who see nothing, feel nothing, experience nothing. If that is you, don't worry. It means your mind is not yet able to perceive your energetic experiences. But you can just go through the motions, enjoying the experience as a moment of calm. You can invite your mind to notice one thing about your inner landscape. You can fake it until you make it. Imagine what you think you would be perceiving and describe it to yourself. And if you continue to draw a blank, make sure to do the "Porcupine Reset" (pages 102–3) and "Flip Your Halos" (pages 104–6) to encourage your gatekeeper to relax its vigilance.

Some people don't remember their dreams, but they still find it worthwhile to sleep. So I invite you to enter the streams and let your body get the benefits while your mind evolves to allow your perceptions in.

MEET THE ENERGY STREAMS

Your body and field are part of a massive moving energy weave that creates and maintains your form. The strands of this weave are not all identical — each has its own vibration and purpose and influence on your overall creation, just as different strands give a woven fabric color and texture.

This weave of energies is echoed by your circulatory system. You have veins and arteries carrying blood into and out of the heart, as well as a vast network of capillaries that spread the life-giving blood, carrying oxygen and nutrients to support the workings of each organ and tissue in your body. Can you hear or feel or just imagine this whole network of your blood circulating in your body?

Your energies have a similar distribution system. These have been mapped in a number of traditions. You may have heard about meridians, *nadis*, energy channels, or pathways. But don't worry about calling up what you've learned before.

The Guided Visits to these streams of energy flowing through your physical and energetic being will help you make your own, more direct relationships to these energies.

As you know, streams are more than just water flowing in channels — they are whole ecosystems that allow waters, and the life-forms that live in them, to spread, travel, and feed the planet.

By the same token, your *energy streams* carry and distribute various kinds of energy and serve many purposes in the co-creation of your energetic weave. These individual types of energy can be found traveling via certain pathways in your body, but there are all kinds of byways and tributaries linking them within the whole system of streams. And the energy carried there is not limited to the banks of the stream, just as the water in an actual river seeps out or evaporates and travels beyond its limits.

Each energy stream is more than a closed system moving inside your body. It is also a part of a cosmic flow that each of us partakes in. Just as rivers interact with oceans, many of your streams are tidal, running stronger with more access to source at high tide, and running with less cosmic force at low tide, twelve hours later.

It is helpful to get to know these core energies directly and learn how to dialogue with them, care for their pathways, and call upon their healing energies as needed.

When Donna Eden calmed the rabid dog in Sausalito, she was not just holding points and sedating his Triple Warmer meridian at a distance. And she wasn't just waving her hands to tell the dog's stream to calm down. She was engaging with the energy stream in that moment in a much more holistic way. She was entering the stream energetically and influencing it, as she had done countless times in her own body, in the process of healing multiple sclerosis and other illnesses.

The gift my Old Chinese Gentleman gave me was the opportunity to explore the energy streams as the energy feeds they are: for our bodies, in the construction of our shared reality, and perhaps in the cosmic scheme of our existence.

If you have studied meridians and the lists of qualities they have been assigned, worked with the points and other outside-in ways of understanding them, do not throw away your knowledge. But perhaps you might want to set it aside, temporarily suspend your beliefs and intellectual knowledge about them, to get to know them directly for what they are.

If I show you a flame, a rock, a body of water, a large chunk of gold, or a tree, you know what they are, not just intellectually, with words and analysis, but directly, as elements of our natural world. You *grok*— know directly and experientially — their energy and nature. You would never use a rock as a substitute for a flame or ask a chunk of gold to produce fruit.

If you don't know meridians the same way, then I am hoping you'll take the time to get to know them as energy streams, as flavors of your being, as strands in the weave of your creation. When you do, the magic of transformation happens, and you can use it to heal yourself and the world.

I don't consider myself an expert on streams or meridians, though I am a longtime visitor. What I have learned is that they don't match the descriptions in books. They are not fixed pathways with dots, like what you see in the diagrams. Instead, like our earth's waterways, they are moving and flowing, waxing and waning, shifting and diverting. And meridian energies are differentiated; they each have their own "flavor." If I want something sour for my salad dressing, I'm going to reach for vinegar or lemon juice, not chocolate syrup or flour. By the same token, each meridian's energies can serve certain purposes better than others.

Below, you will find tracing instructions and Guided Visits to help you get to know the four energy streams of fire element: energizer, yin protector, heart/connection, and choice/discernment. These streams are the most fruitful ones for evolving your gatekeeper. Although I include the names commonly used in English for the meridians and diagrams of the pathways assigned to them, use these as an entry point only: your streams may not follow those pathways or patterns exactly. Tracing each stream is a kind of preliminary practice that familiarizes you with the stream. Then you can shut your eyes to take the Guided Visit.

Read the exercises through. Then, see what happens to your mind and understanding as you encounter these energies more directly. Let it be playtime: you have the rest of your life to get to know the living streams that you are made of.

If you want voice guidance to visit each stream, download MP3s of each at ellenmeredith.com/visits, password: YBSW.

Tracing Energizer Stream (Triple Warmer Meridian)

High Tide: 9 p.m. to 11 p.m.
Element: Fire
Direction: Yang

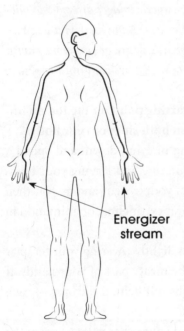

Energizer stream

Figure 6.2. Energizer stream

To begin, bathe your hand in sunlight to activate the cosmic flow.

Then, starting on the back of your hand, at the tip of your fourth (ring) finger, use the flattened palm or fingertips of your other hand to trace straight up the outside of your arm over the elbow (see figure 6.2).

Continue upward to your shoulder, then travel inward across the back of your shoulder and collarbone, up the side of your neck, and beneath your ear. Follow around behind and over your ear, ending at your temple.

Trace this stream on both sides of your body.

Note: Tracing a stream forward (as we just did) helps to support or fortify its flow; tracing it backward helps to calm it or clear it of debris.

Guided Visit: Energizer Stream

The cosmic source of the energizer stream is the sunlight, the enlivening light that animates the life force and warms and illuminates all living beings.

The energizer stream is a place to visit when you need to find safety in your outer reality: your life, your actions, your world. It is also a place to come when you find yourself struggling with your identity in the world or in the eyes of others or when you want to address the various forms of yang gatekeeper reactivity: fight, flight, flood, flutter, fiddle.

The energizer stream helps you to distribute vital qi: it is the stream to turn to when you want to manage stress hormones or immune system responses and mediate between water, or source qi, and fire, or gatekeeping qi.

It is a place to visit to meet with your energetic budget director: to allocate resources, fund certain choices, defund others. And where you can visit when habits keep you from enacting your heart's desire or conscious choice. Also a good place to drop into when dealing with physical immune system symptoms or sluggish immunity.

Trace your energizer flow from its starting point on the fourth finger to its ending point at your temples, on both sides of your body.

Get comfortable where you are sitting or lying down, and spend a few moments just noticing your breath entering and leaving your body. Notice the sensations as the oxygen enters your system and as you then exhale. Notice any sense of movement, vibrancy, tingling, or animation in this body of yours.

Now, cradle your face with both hands, lightly covering your temples with your fingertips and your jaws with the meaty part of your hands. If it's comfortable, let the tips of your thumbs rest behind the base of each ear. Hold like that for several deep breaths.

Then, keeping one hand in place, move your other palm to cover the base of your throat. Hold those two areas for several breaths.

Choose the energizer stream on just one side of your body to explore today. Imagine yourself shrinking down to become a miniature explorer, so you can walk the banks of this stream or even climb into a small boat to travel within it. Let yourself be drawn to whatever entry point calls to you — either the entry point at the tip of your ring finger or another place along the pathway.

Take a moment to notice the flow of your energizer stream. The normal direction of flow is from fingertip upward to your temple. But what is your stream doing? Is the flow steady or choppy? Heading directly upward or swirling against obstacles? Is it a strong flow or weak?

How high is the energy level in the stream bank? What do you notice about the energies? Feel their color, rhythm, personality, how they move.

For those of you who don't perceive much, don't worry. Just commune with the stream and take soundings at different places along the pathway.

Now, expand your attention to the banks and surroundings. What do you notice about the landscape around your stream?

Slowly travel along the stream, noticing what you can. Pay attention to places where you might want to rest and enjoy the scenery or where you might stop to fish. If you want to ask a question — maybe about your safety, or identity, or anything to do with your immune system — ask the question, throw in a line, and see what you pull up. Are the fish biting today? Just note whatever you pull in, without judgment — you can interpret it later.

Ask the stream what it needs from you, today and over time. Then, just listen. Maybe the stream will speak; maybe a guide will show up to answer. Again, don't judge what you hear, just note it.

If the stream shows you something it needs right now, try to supply it, at least symbolically. You can call on the Universal Supply Team to send in workers or use tapping, pulsing, massage, and gesture to do what you can to improve the stream and the environment that surrounds it. This is just a short bit of work. You can leave the helpers to follow through or return later to do more.

Take a moment to do the "Porcupine Reset" (pages 102–3) while you are in this space. If you don't want to do a full-body version, picture a mini-me version of yourself in the space and use your fingers to complete the motions.

Thank your energizer stream for the visit, as well as whatever guides showed up. Now make your way to an exit point — anyplace along the stream where you can return back to the surface of your awareness.

Take a minute to jot down what you remember about the encounter.

⚭ • ⚭

Tracing Yin Protector Stream
(Circulation/Sex Meridian)

High Tide: 7 p.m. to 9 p.m.
Element: Fire
Direction: Yin

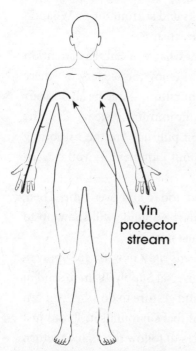

Yin
protector
stream

To start, open your palm to receive moonlight or reach out and imagine grasping the moon in one hand to activate the cosmic flow.

Now, place the fingers of one hand at the outer edge of the opposite nipple. Trace with your fingers up to the front of the shoulder, then down along the inside of the arm and off the middle finger (see figure 6.3).

Yin protector stream runs on both sides of your body. Repeat with the opposite hand on the other side.

Figure 6.3. Yin protector stream (circulation/sex meridian)

Guided Visit: Yin Protector Stream

The cosmic source of the yin protector stream is the moon, aligning you with the pull of the tides, the turning of cycles. It represents the inner knowing reflected in the outer world, as moonlight is a reflection of the sunlight. It illuminates the night, the unknowing, giving the gift of vision in the darkness.

The yin protector stream is a place to come to explore issues of self-protection, particularly relating to your inner sanctity of self, your inner identity. It is a place to come when your heart or inner core feel challenged, when you are reacting to situations with freeze, fog, fade, fatigue, faint, fall apart, fumble, falter, fail, or fibrillate. It is also a place to come when you need to open to others or let go and relax muscles in the body.

This stream is helpful when you have any challenges relating to self-regulation. The physical pathway associated with this stream is the vagus nerve. It is a place to visit when you want to address stage fright, fainting, digestion, reproductive hormones, blood circulation, or other regulation of fluids in your body.

Trace your yin protector stream from beside your nipple to the tip of your middle finger.

Once again, get comfortable and follow your breath as it travels in and out of your body, bringing in oxygen, pausing to let that breath settle, releasing the exhale, and resting empty. Place one hand on your heart and left lung, like you are pledging allegiance or acknowledging that you have been touched by something. Continue to breathe in and out while holding your heart and lung.

Now, place one hand flat on either side of your neck, with your fingertips extending up behind your ear. Let your other hand wander to cover any part of your body that wants the touch and attention right now. Allow those two places to hook up, until you feel something shift or settle or you find yourself taking a deep breath. Continue making other hook-ups you feel you want or need right now.

Imagine yourself shrinking down to become a miniature explorer or just sink your attention down into the stream. Let yourself be drawn to whatever entry point along this stream calls to you.

Stop a moment and listen. What do you hear? Dip your toe or hand into the stream to feel it. What sensations arise for you? Use all your senses, including direct knowing and thought, to get to know this energy stream. If you are comfortable doing so, dip your whole self into the stream, bathing in its energies.

Take a moment to notice the flow of your yin protector stream. The normal direction of flow is from beside the nipple down toward the tip of your middle finger. But what is your stream doing? How is its flow: smooth, choppy, direct, or moving every which way?

How high are the energies in the stream bank? What do you notice about them? Feel their color, rhythm, personality, how they move.

If you find you can't answer any of these questions, don't worry. Just visit the pathway at different places and make connection with the stream.

Your yin protector stream has many underground passages and unseen tributaries. It feeds many of the other streams in your body. If there is another place in your body you instinctively feel needs a stronger connection, hold one hand at any point on your heart protector stream and create a linkage with that other part of your body.

Now, return your attention to the yin protector stream bank and its surroundings. What is the path of this river? How direct or twisty is it? What do you notice about the landscape around it?

If you are having trouble perceiving, flip your halos (pages 104–6) and see if that helps. Draw hearts over your heart.

Slowly travel along the stream, noticing what you can about it. Keep your eye out for caves or sanctuaries. This stream protects the inner sanctity of your self, so there may be places along its path that will take you deep into the source of your being. If you see a cave or sanctuary, ask for permission from the keeper of the space to enter it. Take some time to explore it. Ask if there are teachers or guides here to help you with your explorations.

Ask the stream what it needs from you, today and over time. As before, just listen. Maybe the stream will speak; maybe a guide will show up to answer. Don't judge what you hear, just note it.

If the stream asks for or shows you something it needs right now, try to supply it, at least symbolically. Or call on the Universal Supply Team to send in workers. You can leave the team with instructions and return later to follow through or update your instructions.

Now emerge anywhere along the stream. Place your hand over your heart and lungs again. Pledge allegiance to your heart and the inner sanctity of your self. Thank your yin protector stream and whatever guides showed up for the visit.

Take a minute to jot down what you remember about the encounter.

∽ • ∾

Tracing Heart/Connection Stream (Heart Meridian)

High Tide: 11 a.m. to 1 p.m.
Element: Fire
Direction: Yin

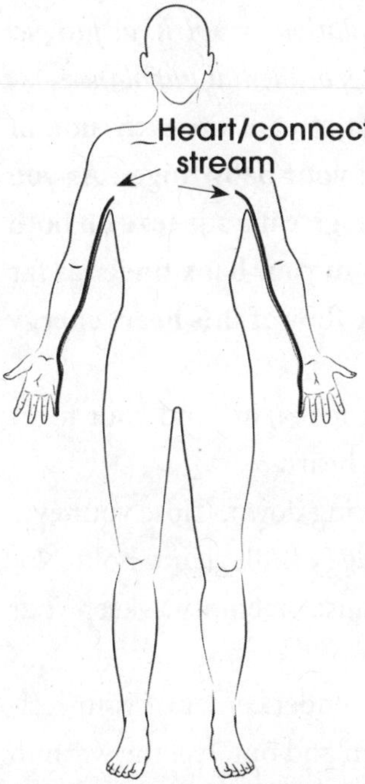

Figure 6.4. Heart/
connection stream
(heart meridian)

Activate the cosmic flow by placing your hand on the heart of the Divine or the heart of mother earth, however you imagine doing that.

Then, place one open hand underneath the opposite armpit in alignment with your little finger. Using your palm or fingertips, trace straight down the inside edge of the arm and off the little finger (see figure 6.4). Heart/connection stream runs on both sides of your body. Switch hands and do this on the other side.

If you wish, you can give your fingertip a squeeze and pull the energy out beyond your fingertips, to arm's length.

Tracing this stream forward (as just described) helps to support or fortify its flow; tracing it backward helps to calm or clear it of debris.

Note: With the heart/connection stream, always trace it forward two to three times after you have traced it backward, to support proper flow and removal of any energetic debris you might have released with the backward tracing.

Guided Visit: Heart/Connection Stream

The cosmic source for the heart/connection stream is the heart of the Divine, heart of mother earth, or heart of truth.

This is the place to come to take refuge, to renew your allegiance to what you hold dear, to find sanctuary, to explore your feelings, to encounter your Wiser Self, and to listen to the dictates of your spirit.

Similarly, it is a place to visit when you are experiencing electrical disturbances; issues with rhythm, pulse, blood circulation, or spirit; or fatigue, insomnia, dizziness, anxiety, love woes, stuttering, or mental imbalances.

Trace the path of your heart/connection stream on each side of your body, from your armpit to the inside of your baby finger. As you trace the stream off the tip of your little finger, give it a squeeze on both sides of the nail, then draw the stream out from your baby finger as far as your tracing arm will reach, to support the flow of this heart energy out into the world.

Start by doing a "Porcupine Reset" (pages 102–3) around your heart organ and tracing hearts over your anatomical heart.

Get comfortable where you are sitting or lying down. Close your eyes and place your hand on your heart, in the Pledge of Allegiance hold. Notice your breath entering; pause; release; and pause on empty...keep your attention here for at least three breaths...

Feel your hand protecting your heart, this tender center of your feelings and home for your spirit. As you breathe in and out, feel the warmth from your hand reaching down to your heart and cradling it. Your hand is a loving sun, nourishing this home for your spirit. Sink your attention down into the heart itself. Feel or imagine the rhythm of your heart beating, the blood pumping in and out.

Now move your hand over to the entry point for your heart/connection stream, under your arm. Cradle this heart/connection stream entry point with your palm and connect in with it, as you did with your heart. Does it also have a rhythm or beat?

Now, return to any point along that stream where you feel called to enter. Allow yourself to shrink in size or else sink your attention down to enter this stream of connection. Take a moment to just feel the flow and notice what you find there.

If you are *visual*, look around you.

If you are more *tonal*, or sound oriented, listen.

If you are more *digital*, or perceiving with your brain, listen to what thoughts arise for you.

If you are *kinesthetic*, or sensing, pay attention to what you are feeling as you enter this stream.

Now, explore what you find here. What is the flow of this energy? Is it moving or still, warm or cool, steady or faltering? What is this place you find yourself in? Are you alone, or are others here with you?

Ask the stream what it wants you to know. And if you wish, tell your heart stream something you wish for it to know.

Your heart is your refuge, the home for your soul. What needs to be built here to better house your spirit? To keep you safe? Invite any guides to come advise you, and if you wish, invite the Universal Supply Team to bring what is needed to create the perfect sanctuary for you here, a place you can come to whenever you want to hang out, take refuge, be protected.

You can evolve this sanctuary over time, as needed, but place some talisman or sign here that marks it as yours. If the space is ready for you, enter the sanctuary for a moment and craft a prayer of thanks to the Universal Supply Team, the guides, and your heart stream for giving you this refuge. If it is not ready to be entered, craft your prayer of thanks and bless the refuge, perhaps drawing a five-pointed star and circle to balance and sanctify it.

Now, return your hand to your heart, in the Pledge of Allegiance hold, and find a place along the stream to exit. Follow your breath in and out for three deep inhales and exhales, allowing each out breath to lift you from the stream and return you to your everyday awareness.

Open your eyes, and take a moment to jot down what you experienced.

∞ • ∞

Tracing Choice/Discernment Stream (Small Intestine Meridian)

High Tide: 1 p.m. to 3 p.m.
Element: Fire

Direction: Yang

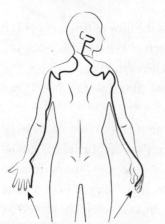

Choice/discernment stream

Figure 6.5. Choice/
discernment stream
(small intestine meridian)

Activate this cosmic stream by holding out both hands and feeling your air roots or earth roots.

Starting at the little finger, use your palm or fingertips to trace straight up the outside of the opposite arm to your shoulder (see figure 6.5). Drop your hand back onto your scapula, then trace up to the base of your neck. Continue up the side of your neck, turn inward to your cheekbone, and then trace back to the opening of your ear.

Repeat this with the other hand on the opposite side of your body.

Note: it is not necessary to trace the exact zigzag path in figure 6.5 if you are using your palm or several fingertips.

Tracing this stream backward clears and calms it; tracing it forward, as we just did, strengthens and supports it.

Guided Visit: Choice/Discernment Stream

The cosmic source for the choice/discernment stream is the web of connections, the swarm of all-knowing from which you choose and activate individual strands to create the story line of your life. Reach out to your air roots or down into your earth roots to access this source.

This is the stream to visit when you are trying to sort out your experience, when you have some choice you need to make or problem to solve, or when you are trying to find your own truth. This stream gives you access to your gut knowing.

The choice/discernment stream helps you to sort truth from untruth, pure from impure. It is a great place to visit when you are having trouble trusting your own judgment. It is also a place to visit when your digestion (literal or figurative) is challenged and you aren't gleaning the nutrients from your food or experiences.

Fire is about fueling action, so visits here can help you not only to choose but also to recognize concrete actions or steps you can take to set choices in motion.

Trace your choice/discernment stream on each side of your body, from baby finger to the front of your ear.

Close your eyes and get comfortable. Place one hand on your gut with your thumb covering your belly button and the rest of the hand over your small intestine, which snakes around that center part of your pelvic region.

Watch your breath enter and release. Now think about something you're trying to sort out, some choice you need to make, or problem you need to solve, or some situation in which you're trying to find your own truth. Feel into your gut. What sensations arise there as you bring this issue to mind?

Leaving one hand on your gut, bring the other hand up to cradle the side of your face, placing your middle fingertip at the opening of your ear. This is a good way to activate your choice/discernment stream, to think about choices, and to listen to your truth.

Imagine you're shrinking down to become a small explorer or drop your consciousness into this stream anywhere along its pathway.

Using any or all of your senses, what do you perceive? Are the energies loud or quiet, strong or weak? Are they harmonious or jangled? Are they moving, or are they relatively still? If you perceive movement, is that movement rhythmic or irregular? If you find stillness, is it restful, or does it feel like you're clogged?

Now explore the pathway of the stream. What are the flora and fauna living there? If you can't picture this, if you're not getting anything, just let your imagination supply answers. Make it be a fantasy trip. It's OK.

The flora and fauna that you find living here — are they healthy? What is the ecosystem in this place? What might help it flourish?

Just ask the stream what it needs in order to be healthy and flourish. It might be something really weird; don't censor your answers. Invite any guides to join you in this place to discuss what you can do to help this stream to thrive. Remember, you can bring in the Universal Supply Team if there's work that you'd like them to do here.

This is a great place to come to discern your gut truth, to make choices, and even to initiate actions. Ask the stream and whatever guides are there to give you input on the situation you brought to mind at the beginning of this journey into the choice flow.

Stay open to hints, direct guidance, and even significant silence. Just gather what's offered and don't push for yes/no answers or definitive instructions. Be open to whatever form truth wants to take in this place at this time.

Since this stream is a form of fire energy, it supports the movement of choice into action. Ask your gut stream: *What are one or two concrete actions you can take over the next while to signal your choice and put things into motion?* If you'd like, make up a gesture that encapsulates your choice or knowing, so that you can reanimate it and revisit it over time using that gesture.

If your focus is on the organ of your small intestine itself, experiment with what helps the stream to move or calm its movement, if needed. Use the hand that's holding your gut to give the organ a rhythm and pace, like a conductor giving a beat to the orchestra. This is a good thing to do. If you can't hear your truth or if your thoughts are jangled, giving a rhythm or beat to the organ itself sometimes helps move the stream that feeds it as well.

Now take a moment to thank the stream and the guides for any insights or clues you've received on this visit. Resolve to stay open to additional guidance and commit to recognizing signs over the next few weeks as this stream brings you into greater awareness of what will nourish you.

Leaving one hand on your gut, move your other hand to cover your heart, and thank your heart/connection, yin protector, and energizer streams for supporting this fourth fire stream, your choice stream, in helping you to hear and enact your truth.

When you are ready, watch your breath enter and let your exhale extend in a long, sustained release, allowing it to catch at the back of your throat as it exits. It's what Donna Eden calls a Darth Vader breath. *Acchhhh.* Then lift your hands off your body and open your eyes.

Take a moment to jot down what you experienced and want to remember.

⚭ • ⚭

EVOLVING YOUR GATEKEEPER

Evolving your gatekeeper is first and foremost a relationship-building task. It is not enough to just calm, calm, calm, reset, reset, reset energies. At some point, your gatekeeper needs to learn that you will show up and really make choices that support you. You become the parent you need and perhaps didn't quite get while growing up.

Here is a short list of ways to evolve your gatekeeper:

- Bring consciousness — show up.
- Listen to and learn from your body. Symptoms and reactivity are a communication, not misbehavior.
- Speak your gatekeeper's language.
- Understand the benefit of working directly with energies (versus focusing on specific forms and outcomes).
- Tap into your natural positive motivation.
- Tune in to inner guidance to give your gatekeeper goals and visions to work toward that align with your deeper truth.

- Calm, clean up, and rebuild stronger by addressing safety, identity, habits, and distribution of energies.
- Bring in radiance, your gatekeeper's cosmic partner.
- Entrain to healthy, positive group gatekeepers (page 95).
- Do this work with joy!

Chapter Seven

Ground and Center in a Changing World

Melanie, Jill, and their two dogs took refuge from Covid-19 in a sweet cottage in a rural area of Oregon. They chose to focus their energy on connecting back into mother nature, rather than feeling locked down or limited by the changes in their work and life brought on by the pandemic. And they found themselves deepening into this new, grounded lifestyle, grateful that they had been forced to make a change.

And then wildfire swept through their corner of the state, destroying the small piece of the planet they had befriended and forcing them to evacuate. After a stressful several days away, they returned and were relieved to discover their cottage still standing, but horrified that their beloved new home now sat in a stinky, gutted landscape, charred past recognition.

I'm not trying to scare you — though I admit I'm scaring myself by retelling this story! Instead, I want to point out that many of us, despite our best plans and intentions, are being asked to change our outer circumstances or to find inner resources in the face of unexpected and sometimes undesirable twists in our plots.

How can we learn to ground, find peace, put down roots, and feel safe in a rapidly changing and less predictable world?

Melanie and Jill turned to spiritual practices, including meditation, and found solace in their awareness of the parts of life that are eternal within. This was an excellent choice.

But to support that, it was useful for them to have some additional understandings and energy medicine tools to help them reground and navigate their changes.

We tend to think of *grounding* as simply sending roots down into the earth, like a tree. But in energetic terms, it is more multifaceted than that. Let's unpack the concept of grounding a bit.

First, it is pretty much impossible to ground your body or mind if your energies are scattered and disconnected. *Centering* is what you do to gather your mind and attention and ground them in the here and now.

Second, think about grounding in terms of a grounding wire that wicks off excess energy and returns it to the earth. Without such grounding, electricity can back up and short out an entire house. A number of years ago, we hired an electrician to sink a new grounding wire for our house. He told me that over the years he had been doing that work, the earth had become supersaturated with electricity, and grounding rods now needed to be much longer than before, to reach down to a place that could handle the excess energy. Talk about symbolic!

We need the energetic equivalent of that grounding rod to be able to safely *release* the energies we don't need in a way that doesn't supersaturate our environment or the earth itself.

Third, a tree is grounded by its root system. When a tree sends down roots, it is reaching out to pull in water and nutrients via multiple conduits. Although individual roots can be linked to individual trees, the underground root system is interwoven in a communication system that not only cares for the individual tree but distributes resources to the collective forest.

Furthermore, the tree root system that sustains the life of the tree also communicates via the mycelium, a fungal network that is part of nature's ability to break down matter to mulch the soil. Thus, the force of decay and the force that creates new life work together to maintain the health of the forest. Melanie and Jill were consoled by recognizing this dance between breakdown and new life, destruction leading to new possibilities, as they worked through their feelings of loss and displacement.

Rooting is everything we do to find and assimilate nourishment, beyond just seeking out good nutrition. It also entails cooperating in communication networks that nourish us and help us balance new growth with the decay of the old forms. How can we find healthy affiliations, connections, and nourishment? How can we learn to metabolize that nourishment and also understand our place in the ecology of life-forms?

Fourth, tree roots also *anchor* the tree in the soil. A tree has multiple anchors that ground it, not a single large taproot working alone. When you think of a boat anchor, on the other hand, it keeps the boat safely in harbor while still allowing some drift and movement. How can we find anchors that give us stability in multiple directions, like tree roots, but also flexibility, like a boat anchor that keeps us in range of our fellow beings, our sources of nourishment? Conscious anchoring is an art form!

Taken together, the four *grounding skills* of centering, release, rooting, and anchoring give us security, orientation, and flexibility to change.

This is a particularly crucial skill set to develop now. About fifteen years ago my inner teachers announced that the electromagnetics of the earth were fluctuating. Today north and south are no longer energetically the fixed poles that we used to know. And the energetic heartbeat of the earth, what scientists call the Schumann resonances, is fluctuating as well. At the time the Councils told me about the shift, they said that not only is life on planet earth going to be a bit more of a bucking bronco ride but also the guardians of the planet have set up a stabilized shelf, eight feet below the surface of the earth, where if we do send down taproots we can get a steadier energetic feed. The exercise "Earth Dock–Sky Dock" (available in my book *The Language Your Body Speaks* and on my YouTube channel at youtu.be/yO3fybT14PM) is designed to help you reground using this "earth dock" and other more stable anchors.

The protocol offered on pages 88–92, "Anchoring in the Stabilizing Sphere," is also a great way to create your own "earth" to anchor and ground in. In the following pages, I offer still more tools and techniques to support you in this important work.

In terms of your health and emotional well-being, when you have faulty grounding:

- Your gatekeeper sounds the alarm and triggers reactivity on many levels of your being.

- Your energy flow gets distorted, creating irregular energies that can interfere with the work of your body.
- Energies get backed up in your body and mind, causing disruption.
- Your body releases stress hormones that put your energy to work keeping you safe. This hijacks your ability to heal, build new tissue, think clearly, or experience life on your own terms.
- Nourishment (of all kinds) becomes more difficult to absorb.
- Your body and mind lose their ability to hear your inner guidance system.
- Energy testing and even chemical testing become unreliable.
- If it continues, it can cause chronic imbalance, illness, burnout, and shutdown.

Turning this around, I would say that when you cultivate grounding in all its dimensions, you are deeply supporting your health and well-being from the inside out.

CENTERING: THE SACRED BATON OF THE SELF

Lynn came for an energy medicine session because her hands and feet were itchy, sore, and driving her crazy. I was trying to get her hands and feet to show me what they needed when I heard my Councils say, "It's not in the extremities; look at her sacred baton of the self."

I had never heard this term before, but I saw in my mind's eye a baton, like the ones used in relay races, only made of energies. And it was as if a whole new/old room had opened in my mind. I just *knew* this place, the meaning of what they were asking me to do.

Your *sacred baton of the self* is your energetic spine, a central corridor that runs along your physical spine and is the core you center into and from, ground into and from. It is the part of your self that is passed from lifetime to lifetime and that forms the energetic ground on which you build your body and life.

Sometimes we get to know things piece by piece, through experience, and sometimes knowing comes to us whole, even if we spend the rest of our lives unpacking its implications and what it means, finding proofs or techniques that allow us to work with it. This came to me whole, *and* I have spent the last thirty-three-plus years figuring out different ways to work with it, developing a practice I came to call *Energy Chiro*.

Your energetic spine is a place where you can access your deep knowing and your energetic truth. It is certainly a rich place to visit for information, to dig for gold, and to clean and clear in order to allow communications to flow throughout your body.

With Lynn, I asked her to lie on her stomach, and I took a tour of her sacred baton of the self. I worked like a dental hygienist, clearing and cleaning energies in and around her vertebrae and in that whole central corridor that opened up to my vision.

I could almost *hear* what needed to happen. It felt like one of those old-fashioned telephone operator exchanges, where all the calls had to go through a central switchboard. Only her lines were not properly plugged in. Some were just dangling, some were in the wrong places, and others were crossed. So I let the wisdom in my hands and her energetic spine itself guide the work.

And when Lynn turned over onto her back, she was a different person! She was completely centered and grounded, present, clear; and not only were her hands and feet comfortable, but, in her words, they felt "inspired"!

I'm not the only person to discover this magical place. It is at the center of many traditions and practices. Think for a moment about what you've got in that region. On the physical level you have the vertebrae of your spine, which allow you to be upright and provide structure. You have disks that are designed to allow flexibility of movement and provide cushioning from stress. Your spine is a central communication pathway for your nerves, which spread out from there to all your organs and extremities. You have cerebrospinal fluid, which facilitates communication between your brain and body, and you have a blood supply that fuels the work of your brain and nervous system. It is not rocket science to figure out that this physical center would play a role in any illness or disease.

Energetically, what sits in there is a central corridor that links all your streams. (I call the two streams of this corridor *conception* and *comprehension*.) You have your energetic grid, a matrix of energies laid down by your soul, like a foundation to build your body and life on. You have your primary chakras, energy distribution systems that feed your body and facilitate exchange with the world. And the energetic spine, together with the chakras, serves as a central library where you store the energetic experiences from all your lifetimes. It is the interface between your body and soul.

If this is too woo-woo for you, then you can just focus on the fact that all of the communications of the body travel through the spine to get where they are going. It is the Grand Central Station of your being, and if the traffic flow through there is disturbed or blocked, then no one can get where they are trying to go!

Try the following three activities to explore and get to know your energetic spine.

Tracing Conception Stream (Central Vessel)

Element: Air
Direction: Bidirectional

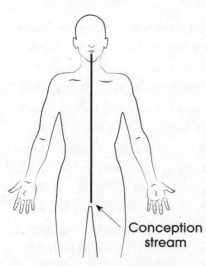

Conception stream

Figure 7.1. Conception stream (central vessel)

If possible, touch the earth to activate the cosmic stream. Otherwise, just attune your hand to the earth. Then feel the air around you, buoying you.

Place both hands at the base of your torso in front, on your pubic bone, and bring them straight up the front of your body to your bottom lip, as if you were zipping up a zipper (see figure 7.1).

From here, the conception stream dips back to join the comprehension stream at the back of your throat in a burst of light.

In this Eden Energy Medicine exercise, if you want to keep yourself zipped up energetically, meaning less vulnerable to the influence of others, you can lock the zipper in place with a twisting motion at the top.

To clear, trace the stream downward. To reinstate or reinforce it and strengthen your protections, zip upward. Always end this tracing with an upward zip.

Tracing Comprehension Stream (Governing Vessel)

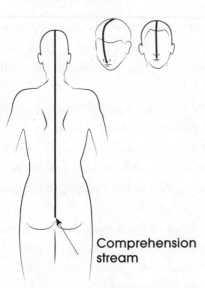

Comprehension stream

Figure 7.2. Comprehension stream (governing vessel)

Open your palm to the heavens and soak in energy from the sky or your soul's star to activate the cosmic stream.

Place one palm facing your tailbone and trace with your hand or fingers straight up your spine as high as you can (figure 7.2).

Then, reach over your shoulder, connecting into the line you've drawn (if you can't reach, use your imagination), and use that hand to trace the energy the rest of the way up your spine, over the centerline of the back and top of your head, down the center of your face, over your nose, to your top lip.

From here the comprehension stream dips to the back of your throat at the base of your skull with a burst of light.

If you wish to lock this back zip up, to protect your mind and back from undue influence, mime turning the key and stashing it in your pocket. Trace this stream backward to clear and forward to strengthen.

Guided Visit: Conception and Comprehension Streams

The cosmic source of the conception vessel is the earth herself and the air surrounding her.

The cosmic source of the comprehension vessel is the sky — or you can use your soul's star (the star with your name on it) if you wish.

Although we usually trace them both upward from the root, in their circular microcosmic orbit, the conception corridor arises from the earth, and the comprehension corridor descends from the sky. The energies mix in their shared orbit, traveling in both directions.

You actually have three cosmic sources meeting in the energetic spine, since it is also the seat of the grid, whose cosmic source is the soul. These three cosmic sources — earth, sky, and the soul — source your three selves: Earth Elemental Self, Talking Self, and Wiser Self.

Conception vessel is the place where you take in energies and give birth both literally and figuratively to ideas, projects, knowing. This is the birthplace, the core, of your energies. It is a good place to visit when you want to investigate what is influencing you from without and within. It is also a good place to plant affirmations and intentions. Any health issues affecting your midline can be explored here.

Comprehension vessel is the stream that connects most directly to your brain, so it is a great place to come when you need to formulate understanding, conscious awareness. But don't worry about getting clear, direct answers — just know that if you put in the request, your librarians will work on it in the background, until they can fulfill it. It is also a good stream to visit when you have physical issues with your spine or in your brain or with connecting brain and body. (For these types of issues you may also want to visit the distribution/bladder stream; see page 227.)

Trace your conception stream from pubic bone to bottom lip, then your comprehension stream from sacrum to top lip.

Get comfortable where you are sitting or lying. Shut your eyes. Place your hands on your midline and notice your breath coming in, and releasing, coming in, and releasing …

Tune in to your energetic spine, however you want to picture it. This is the sacred baton of your self — your energetic core. Greet your sacred baton and thank it for carrying your life force into this life.

Feel both of the streams you traced flowing upward from your root to nourish your front and back. Feel their connection and interaction as they meet at your *power point* (the base of your skull, where it meets your spine) and form a circular flow, a *microcosmic orbit*, moving in both directions around your core, bathing your spine with energy, carrying information in both directions.

Let's take a few minutes to explore your conception vessel in front — the place where you take in energies and give birth, both literally and figuratively, to new life, ideas, projects, knowing. Tap with your fingers up and down this stream, to activate its flow.

Shrink down so you can enter the stream or sink your awareness down into it, wherever along its pathway you are drawn to do so.

What do you notice about the energies of this central corridor at your core? If you want to see the space as a stream, what do you notice about its flow, contents, health? And if you don't see it as a stream, what kind of space or environment are you experiencing as you attune to this part of your being?

Don't worry about what you do or don't perceive. Just notice what shows up as you commune with this space.

Ask the space what it needs from you. And ask if there are guides in this place to help you heal or thrive more fully.

If you can see a way to clear or refresh the stream, invite the Universal Supply Team to come help you set that work in motion.

Because this is the birthplace, the core, of your energies, is there a seed you'd like to plant or a request you'd like to submit to your Wiser Self? If so, plant or submit it now.

We are going to temporarily leave this stream and travel into the comprehension stream, which runs up the back of your body. To get there, you can either travel through your body or emerge to the surface and find a place to enter the comprehension stream on your back.

If you wish, place one hand on your sacrum and the other at the base of your skull where it meets your spine, your power point. Hold this for at least three deep breaths.

What do you notice about your comprehension stream? What is the flow like? How does this place feel different from where you just visited? How is it similar?

Travel along the path of this stream, noticing where the flow is easy and where it seems to be obstructed or less smooth. What is your feeling as you commune with this place? What thoughts arise?

Ask if there are guides here to help you find your way. If there is something you wish to comprehend, pose a question or put in a request.

When you are ready, travel back around the microcosmic orbit of energies encircling your spine and your sacred baton of the self. Go in whichever direction feels comfortable, traveling the loop a few times to really get the feel of these circulating energy streams. Continue around until you return to the front of your body.

Now, consciously breathe in and out. Use each exhale to rise out of the streams. Bring your attention first to your hands on your body and then to the room around you, and when you are ready, open your eyes.

Take a moment to jot down anything you want to remember from this visit.

∽ • ∽

In conjunction with entering the streams, you can do the following protocol, "Clearing the Sacred Baton of the Self," when you return to the front of your body. Or you can do this protocol on its own. "Clearing the Sacred Baton of the Self" is a variation on a method taught in Eden Energy Medicine called the "Hopi Healing Technique." While that is usually taught to practitioners as a pain reliever, this version, with energetic laser lights and anchoring, can be a powerful self-help tool for spine clearing and anchoring/grounding.

Protocol: Clearing the Sacred Baton of the Self

This exercise can be done on yourself, up the front of your body, or for another person, traveling up the back of their spine. Instructions here are for doing it on yourself. It can clear clogged energies, relieve pain, center you, and help anchor you.

1. Bend your fingers as if you are playing the piano. Keeping the fingers bent, place one hand on one side of your pubic area and the other hand on the other side. (If your hands were in the back, your fingers would be on either side of your spine, just adjacent to the bony processes, those spinal arms that extend from your vertebrae.)

2. Activate your fingers as if they are streaming colored laser lights. Send that energy through your body and out the back, cleaning and clearing and renewing the energies of your spine and opening any clogged or congested areas. Tune in to see what you perceive about the area. Is there congestion? Is the energy able to travel straight through, or does it get diverted? What do your finger lights encounter as they try to pass through this area?

    Make this a gentle invitation to your spine to open. You can use your inhales to attune with the area and the exhales to pulse the laser lights out your fingers, using the vibrations of light and color to lovingly untangle and open up your spinal energies.

3. As the lights exit the back of your spine, invite them to extend and anchor somewhere wholesome, and notice where they anchor. Let the lights themselves, in their wisdom, seek these anchoring points rather than trying to assign them landing places. The anchor might be somewhere in nature. It might be inside the hands or hearts of loving guides. It might be in something you feel gives you strength and nourishment. Don't worry about the physical logistics of this anchoring. Energy can anchor through resonance with like-spirited places or beings.

4. Now, move your hands upward along the midline of your body, and place them just above where your hands have been positioned, and again send the laser lights gently through the front and back corridors, clearing space and opening your energies. Don't force it. Let them emerge and seek a wholesome anchor.

5. Move your hands upward along the spine again to a position in your solar plexus area, just above where they were sitting before, and again send the laser lights in to clear a path through your core. Once more pulse these lights all the way through, then send them further to anchor somewhere and note where they land.

6. Keep moving your hands up along the midline, stopping in turn at the rib cage, between your breasts, then on your upper chest beside your lungs, at each position directing your laser lights through to open a pathway and clear obstructions, gently and with a spirit of opening and invitation. Send them further to anchor and observe where they land.

7. Now move your hands once again upward, along your throat, still in line with your spinal processes. Breathe in. On the exhale, send the laser lights in to clear out any congested energies in your spine and neck, using the vibrations of the colors along with your exhale to softly open and release tensions, constrictions, blockages. And as you inhale and exhale, continue sending the lights further until they emerge in back, seeking safe harbor to anchor in.

8. To finish this exercise, feel into your spinal core and sense the anchors you have moored in safe harbors. Place one hand on your heart and the other hand on your solar plexus. Thank your sacred baton of the self for its gifts.

☞ • ☜

Your energetic spine has several particularly potent access points through which you can influence the larger energetic flows in your body. To get your central switchboard working better and facilitate communications in your spine, you can hook up these access points using the "Zigzag Hook-Up" protocol below.

Protocol: Zigzag Hook-Up

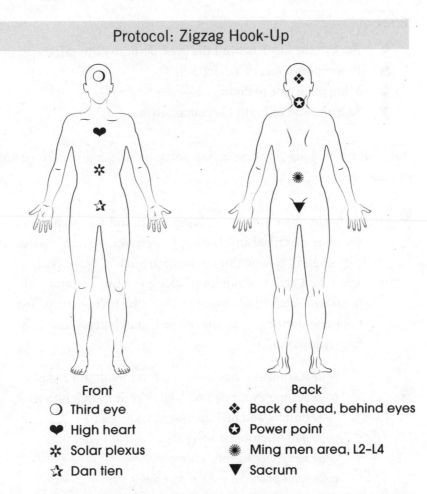

Front
- ○ Third eye
- ♥ High heart
- ✳ Solar plexus
- ☆ Dan tien

Back
- ❖ Back of head, behind eyes
- ✪ Power point
- ✺ Ming men area, L2–L4
- ▼ Sacrum

Figure 7.3. Key energy access points on the sacred baton of the self

The sacred baton of the self has several key energy access points (see figure 7.3). From top to bottom, they are:

Front of Body:

- ○ **Third eye:** the seat of the Wiser Self
- ♥ **High heart:** home for your soul
- ✳ **Solar plexus:** core of your identity
- ☆ **Dan tien:** access to your authentic self

Back of Body:

- ❖ **Back of the head, behind the eyes:** point to calm gatekeeper
- ✪ **Power point:** seat of Talking Self
- ✳ **Ming men:** gate of destiny, doorway to depth
- ▼ **Sacrum:** seat of Earth Elemental Self

You will be hooking up these access points in a zigzag pattern passing through your body.

1. To begin, trace your conception vessel and comprehension vessel as described in "Tracing Conception Stream" (pages 150–51) and "Tracing Comprehension Stream" (page 151).
2. Then do a series of hook-ups along the two pathways. Do them with both hands together or, if that isn't possible, first hold one position, then the other. Using flattened hands or fingertips, connect:

- your *sacrum* to your *dan tien.* (If you want, you can place your palm on your dan tien, hook your thumb into your belly button, and pull up toward your head.)
- your *dan tien* to your *ming men.*
- your *ming men* to your *solar plexus.*
- your *solar plexus* to your *power point.*
- your *power point* to your *high heart.*
- your *high heart* to the *back of your head.*
- your *back of your head* to your *third eye.* To do this, flatten one hand on your forehead and also use your full flattened hand on the back of your head, behind your eyes. (This hold is great to calm your gatekeeper.)
- the *back of your head* to your *high heart.*

To complete the hook-up sequence, leave one hand on your high heart and use the other to hold hands with the Divine (page 107), however you picture doing that.

3. Now take three deep breaths with long exhales while holding one hand on your high heart and the other on your solar
   plexus.

∽ • ∽

Grounding is a rich topic. We've just taken a deep dive into centering in and strengthening your energetic core. In chapter 8, "Ground in Your Inner Wisdom," we will explore the other three dimensions of this crucial skill set for building resilience and navigating change: *release, anchoring,* and *rooting.*

ᖆ Chapter Eight ᖆ

Ground in Your Inner Wisdom

For those of us who grew up in this evidence-based, outside-in culture, inner wisdom can seem like a vague and unreliable resource. But in fact, grounding your energies to stay anchored within change requires that you establish some kind of true north within yourself. Without it, there is nothing reliable to navigate by. To get to inner wisdom, though, it is not always as easy as just asking your inner self for insight. Most of us have been socialized with too many layers of distortion to get clear guidance right away. It's helpful to explore more fully how to get your energies grounding better, via release, anchoring, and rooting.

RELEASE

Before you can take in a breath, you need to release what is in your lungs. Before you can eat another meal, your body needs to process and release all the food you ate at your last meal. Before you can take in someone's love, you need to make space for it in your heart and mind.

The art of clearing and releasing energies is a crucial skill for being able to navigate change. If we can't let go of the old, we can't make space for something new. When Melanie and Jill's beloved forest burned down, part of what allowed them to move past the shock and grief was to recognize that mother nature needs to clear the ground to support new growth.

As someone who processes things tonally, through sound, and as someone whose primary element is earth, release did not come naturally to me. Tonals have "sticky brains." We have trouble unhearing things and moving on. Earths can be collectors, because you never know when you'll need something. And many of my early bouts with illness had an element of challenge in this realm: difficulty clearing my mind, difficulty letting go and entering sleep, difficulty releasing energy buildup in my head. Difficulty letting go of obsessive thoughts, difficulty getting myself to move and let go of pent-up stresses.

So let's just say this is a topic dear to my heart. I have found that it is useful to look at what motivates you to let something go. Think about the little kid who has grabbed Mom's car keys and won't let go. How can you motivate that kid to give over the keys? Usually by offering a substitute. Some other shiny toy Mom doesn't need right now.

And when a stressed-out dog or cat is cowering or hissing, how do we get them to release their stance? Maybe by crooning loving reassurances, by giving them time to release, by backing off.

෨ Play with It! ෨

How comfortable are you with letting go, releasing? How well do you digest and release your food? How well do you let go of a disagreement or difficult interaction? How well do you move on after an experience? How much do you hold on to that interferes with your present choices?

On the physical level, how much do electrical activity and stress chemicals hang around in your body? And on the mental level, how long do emotions hang around in your mind, interfering with your ability to meet the present moment with a relatively clear mind and neutral energy?

Tune in to how each of these feels in your body or mind, right now.

Now, play around with creating a gesture of release for each of these ways you hold on. Or you might find one general motion that supports both your body and mind to let go.

When I release energy, I like to send it into the Universal Recycling Bin. I grab the energy, pull it out, swing my arms around, and throw it into the bin. That way it doesn't pollute my house, or mother earth, or my immediate environment. As you practice release, consider where you would like to send your excess.

Sometimes, if I don't want to get rid of it, I send it to my energetic off-site storage facility. There the keeper of my excess can send the thoughts or energies back to me if I need them.

Tune in once again to your body and mind. What has shifted with your gesture of release?

◌ • ◌

When I was first working with the energetic spine, my Councils said, "The cleaner your cerebrospinal fluid, the better your body, mind, and spirit can flow." Because of that, I began to check into my spinal fluid periodically, to see how clean it felt, and I also checked the fluid on each client.

Invariably the clients' spinal fluid was murky, filled with what looked like particles that didn't belong. And when someone was actively ill, I could often see it in what their spinal fluid looked like. It gets opaque or discolored and gunky when someone is ill. Turning that around, when your spinal fluid is cloudy, discolored, or gunky, it is highly likely you will fall ill.

Here is a simple exercise I use to help clear the cerebrospinal fluid.

Exercise: Spinal Fluid Screen

With both hands, grab the frame of an imaginary screen that is bigger in size than your physical body. I picture a window screen with a very fine mesh.

Hold the screen up above your head, inhale, and on the exhale, very slowly bring the screen down through your body, capturing impurities and particles that don't belong and filtering your spinal fluid as it goes.

Pause when you need to inhale, then continue moving the screen downward on the exhale until you bring the screen to the ground. I then step beside it, gather up what I have strained from my system, and throw it in the Universal Recycling Bin.

You can also filter your energies from the ground up if that feels more natural for you.

Repeat the process as many times as needed, with ever-finer mesh, until you feel your spinal fluid is sparkling and clear.

∞ • ∞

Often my clients develop muscle pain or fixed thoughts or stuck emotions that just refuse to release. For these situations, I use a technique called "Grab and Walk Away." It may sound crazy, but sometimes it just helps to give a good tug to extricate unwanted energies!

Exercise: Grab and Walk Away

This is wonderful to do for another person (or ask someone to do it for you). Using gesture, grasp the person's muscle tightness, stuck thoughts, or emotions in your hand. Ask them to inhale and then, on the exhale, have them slowly walk away. As they move away from you, hold on to their stress or stuckness tightly (as if you were landing a struggling fish), helping to ease it out of their body and energy field. When they run out of air to exhale, have them stop walking, inhale, then continue walking again on the exhale. Continue the exercise until you have pulled the obstruction all the way out of their energy field.

I put a lot of muscle into this action.

To do "Grab and Walk Away" for myself, I use gesture to tie the stress or blockage to an imagined hook on the wall. Then I inhale and walk slowly away on the exhale, pulling the stressor out of my body and field, as described above. Finally, I remove the energetic stress from the hook and throw it in the Universal Recycling Bin.

∞ • ∞

ANCHORING

Tillie's parents died within a year of each other. She realized it was a big change to become a member of the eldest generation and did some journaling and therapy work to help herself make the transition. But then, in rapid succession, her best friend moved away, her dog also died, and her boss left the company, making her workplace an unfamiliar and far less agreeable environment for her.

She woke up one morning unable to move. She felt as if a freight train had run over her. She told herself she was just reacting to grief and loss. And after a few days, she was up and able to go to work. But her energy didn't fully recover. She was tired all the time and had no energy to try to change things up.

When she asked me for a channeled reading, she expected to be told by her Councils that she just needed to give herself time to process the grief. Instead, they said, "You have lost your anchors and are drifting at sea. You need some new anchors, better stars to navigate by, and you need to learn the art of conscious anchoring." They went on to suggest a number of possible places where she could anchor herself.

I taught her to clear the sacred baton of her self (pages 154–56), suggesting she focus particularly on the anchoring part — where did those lights land? Who was catching them? She decided to do the exercise at least once or twice a day and keep notes on who caught her energies at each place. Then she'd look in her life for where she might experience that energy symbolically.

Her first time through, her lights were caught by a group of children flying kites, a circle of older women sharing wisdom, an officious kind of person who wanted to sort all the lights, her father's spirit, and a fertile field. She was dubious about her Councils' suggested assignment to bring those energies into her life. But she decided to volunteer one afternoon a week at the local YMCA to watch children playing, and she joined a support group of women considering retirement. She did not have a yard in which to plant a garden, but she bought several pots to grow herbs in, and she decided to write a series of letters to her father, thanking him for the gifts she had gotten from him.

I heard back from Tillie two months later. She told me that her energies had returned to normal. She made the anchoring exercise part of her daily routine.

⌒ Play with It! ⌒

Do the protocol on pages 154–56, "Clearing the Sacred Baton of the Self," and this time focus on who or what is catching your colored light energies as you send them down into the earth. Just travel up the energetic spine, letting it show you where it wants to anchor. Let the knowing come to you, rather than trying to call up or assign anchors. At each place along the spine, you can briefly jot down reminders for yourself of what you experienced so you'll remember later.

When you have made one pass, go back through again and try to dialogue with each anchor. Ask them who they are and what they bring you. Ask the energies to show you ways you can know them in your everyday life.

And, if possible, follow through with at least one of the suggestions by taking real or at least symbolic action.

⌒ • ⌒

If your anchors are in place but not necessarily wholesome, you can use "Anchoring in the Stabilizing Sphere" (pages 88–92) to help you evolve your ability to anchor from the inside out. For example, if what anchors your day is reading the news, drinking coffee, pushing yourself to do exercises you hate, then working your way through a to-do list of things you feel you have to do, you can anchor in the stabilizing sphere at the start and/or ending of each day, infusing the sphere with whatever quality or resources you feel you need. This practice will support you energetically to experiment with change in your daily habits. And if your emotional anchors are friends who keep you stuck in old behavior patterns, then anchoring regularly in the stabilizing sphere can give you the inner stability to change those relationships.

Sometimes the people, habits, and places we anchor to are in fact tying us down and keeping us from the activities we need that will give us adequate nutrients. If you have given up flexibility and change in exchange for security, in terms of a pretty fixed universe, you can explore lifestyle activities that pull you out of your routine. Take a drive or walk in beautiful scenery. Vary your routes of travel. Shift your schedule or social commitments. It is helpful to have our muscles of change well warmed up — before change forces itself upon us!

ROOTING, OR NOURISHMENT

We are a lot more like trees than common belief would admit. We share an energetic root system with our fellow beings. We take in nourishment from the sun and water and air and earth around us, which we use to build new tissue, fuel our projects, create new life. Then, when we have used what we can, we return what we don't need to mulch the earth.

When I ask my clients about what nourishes them, they invariably start talking about their literal nutrition: what foods they put in their mouths. And because of the type of clients I have tended to attract, many of them are following a diet that is based on the latest scientific information about what inputs they should have in order to be healthy.

This obsession with inputs in our culture begs the question of what happens to the food when it enters your body or tries to leave again. And it begs the question of whether what you, specifically and individually, need in order to be truly nourished physically, emotionally, and energetically is something scientists can determine and prescribe.

Angie's parents were famous health food advocates. So you can imagine how embarrassing it was for her to have to seek support when her digestive system was in an uproar. She was not able to digest any of the foods she *knew* she should eat. Eden Energy Medicine includes techniques for energy testing foods, asking the body which ones it can handle. At the request of her practitioner, Angie brought in a large selection of foods to energy test. At the end of the session, it turned out that the only two foods Angie's body would accept at that time were full-fat premium ice cream and bacon!

Angie was horrified that her body told her to eat no-no's. But she was desperate, so she agreed to go on a bacon and ice cream diet for the next week and see what would happen. Over that week, her symptoms receded. And after two weeks, her digestion was back in gear, willing and able to digest pretty much anything — as long as she practiced attuned eating and listened to what her body craved and signaled it needed.

When I told this story in a recent class, a number of the students promptly put themselves on a bacon and ice cream diet, though a few attuned to their bodies to figure out their body's specific desires. Many of us get caught in the dietary craziness of our culture, trying to control our inputs rather than seeing food shopping, choosing from bounty, cooking, eating, and self-feeding as part of a larger pattern of nourishment!

Years ago, I edited a publication about malnourishment in young children. There were a number of studies looking at the effects of food inputs and types of feeding and care. The studies showed that the best nourishment was achieved with a combination of feeding plus care. In other words, infants thrive best when they are fed with both nutritious food and love.

This is true of grown-ups as well. We are not just chemical-processing machines. We are in a dynamic exchange with our environment — physically with mother earth, but also energetically with the symphony of life-forms that inhabit this dimension (and beyond). So nourishment is more than a diet, a set of foods. It is everything that you:

- take into your body, mind, and perceptions
- metabolize or process so your body, mind, and spirit can use it
- distribute to the parts of yourself that need it
- use to fuel and support the workings of your body, mind, and spirit
- release or store as appropriate when there is excess or un-needed portions

When you eat a meal, you are eating more than the chemical makeup of the foods on your plate. You are eating the energy of care (or of distraction, deprivation, judgment, or perfectionism). You are eating the atmosphere of nourishment (or desperation or self-criticism or other people's preoccupations).

And if you are then on to your next activity, perhaps the food is just going in one end and coming out the other, without being truly received, appreciated for the gift it is, metabolized, distributed to where it is needed in your body, made available to support your body with the building resources it could supply, and released comfortably and easily when it is not useful.

∽ Play with It! ∽

Ask your digestive system for a name you can call it, as described on page 31. Next, ask it by name to put together a buffet of all the foods, activities, and energies it wants to include on the table for you to choose from. Now, survey the buffet and ask this newly named part of your being which item, if any, it would like now.

Stay open to the possibility that it doesn't want to take in anything right now and instead would like support metabolizing what you took in over the past hour. Or perhaps it wants help with distributing the energies or releasing the excess already in your body.

Then do something to honor that request. What would it be like to treat this newly named part of you like royalty, like the life-giving, life-sustaining being she is? Ask her what she needs from you, not just in terms of inputs but in terms of how she wants to be supported and cared for.

Thank her and continue to dialogue with her over several days or weeks as part of an attuned-nourishment experiment.

∽ • ∽

Babies thrive when we feed them more than formula or breast milk: when they get loved, held, supported, and spoken or sung to as part of the experience of receiving their nutrients. What do you do to love, hold, support, and sing to yourself in providing nourishment for the use of your body, mind, and spirit?

To help you with metabolizing, try the exercise "Metabolizing Eights" (and do it with love!).

Exercise: Metabolizing Eights

In this exercise you trace a figure eight that meets at the center (figure 8.1).

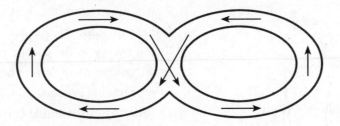

Figure 8.1. Metabolizing eights

Starting at the midline of your body, trace a clockwise circle that moves toward the left outer side of your body, circles forward, and returns to your midline. Then continue with a counterclockwise circle, tracing it out to your right side, and circle forward and toward the left, returning to the midline. Repeat until you feel the energies in that area flowing easily through the center. Once you have learned this pattern of eight, you can move it to center over any part of you that needs support to metabolize. I often trace large metabolizing eights up and down my sacred baton of the self, imagining that I am enfolding myself in a big wave of delicious liquid chocolate.

○○ • ○○

It will not surprise you to hear that the two streams that most support rooting and nourishment are your two earth streams. Enter the yin earth flow I call *nourishment stream* and the yang earth flow I call *embodiment stream* below.

Tracing Nourishment Stream (Spleen Meridian)

High Tide: 9 a.m. to 11 a.m.
Element: Earth
Direction: Yin

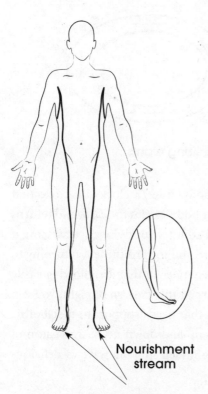

Nourishment
stream

Figure 8.2. Nourishment
stream (spleen meridian)

Reach down into the earth to gather up some of the healing, loving energy in the cosmic part of the nourishment flow to bring to your tracing process.

Starting at the inside corners of each big toenail (nearest your centerline), use your hands or fingertips to trace straight up the insides of your legs, flaring out at your hips and continuing up the front of your body to your armpit (see figure 8.2). Then stroke downward from your armpit along your side halfway down the rib cage.

To clear or calm this flow, trace it backward from its end point at the side of your rib cage to your big toe. To strengthen and support this flow, trace it forward, as described above.

Guided Visit: Nourishment Stream

The cosmic source for this stream is the universal flow from mother earth, a ceaseless energy of nourishment and caring.

This nourishment stream is your inner carer. It brings you the ability to extract nutrients from the earth; to help you metabolize food, experience, and feelings; and to use them to build or repair tissue, strengthen blood, renew cellular energy, and support healing.

This flow is often drained by the energizer stream, so it is important to support and reinforce this stream when stress has depleted you or you are dealing with autoimmune challenges. Metabolizing eights (page 169) are especially helpful to support your nourishment stream.

Trace this flow on both sides of your body, from big toe to the armpit to the side of your rib cage.

Get comfortable where you are lying or sitting down. Close your eyes. Watch your breath come in, assimilate, go out, and empty. Feel this four-part process of taking in, then assimilating the nourishing oxygen, exhaling the carbon dioxide you don't need, and then resting empty...

And as you breathe and participate in this vital process, recognize that the plant kingdom is supplying the oxygen you depend on and that you, in turn, are supplying the carbon dioxide the plants need in order to breathe. Feel this beautiful mutual exchange of life force you participate in each time you breathe, which is so much a part of this earth existence.

Place one hand on the side of your rib cage, over the end point of this stream. Use your other hand to cradle the side of your face, stretching your hand out so the fingertips cover your temples and the base of your hand lightly covers your jawline. Hold for at least three deep breaths.

This stream is a sacred chalice of life-giving earth energy: its base is rooted in the earth itself, its stem rises up through your center to feed your root, and its cup holds and bathes the energies of your organs and torso in its nourishment.

Choose one side of your body to enter the stream, wherever you are drawn along the pathways you just traced. Shrinking down or sinking your attention down into this stream, just feel into it.

Keep one hand on the stream where you entered. What do you notice about where you find yourself? Are you in the lower stem part of the stream or the upper cup part?

What is the flow like? Using all your senses and your noticing mind, just check out this space.

Do you feel at home here? If not, what do you need to make you feel more at home?

Who is home for you here? Invite an inner consoler to join you, here at this stream: Quan Yin, goddess of compassion; Mother Teresa; the Dalai Lama; Glinda the Good Witch; your Councils; your own Wiser Self. Whoever represents that consoling, compassionate energy for you.

If you wish, wrap your arms around yourself in a hug and imagine your consoler also holding you in their arms or in the light of their infinite compassion!

Turn off your mind and just feel the energy of consoling and being consoled in this place.

Now, invite a self that you've been or will be at some time in this life — your two-, or five-, or thirteen-, or thirty-year-old self, or your present or future self — to come into this space with you, to be held and consoled, nourished and made whole, by you and your cosmic consolers. Don't worry about which self to choose — just pick one, because you can always bring another one later. This is a beautiful place to be reassured and mothered, accepted and held, without conditions. No words or knowing or analysis are needed: just you as a mom, as a dad, accepting your young self with compassion, telling this past or future self, "We are all human."

Hold that other version of yourself. Bless them; forgive them; accept them without conditions. If you don't know how, let your cosmic helpers show you the way.

Then use some kind of dipper or cup to bring the energies of this cosmic stream of nourishment to your alternate self: to feed and nourish and anoint them; to strengthen their blood flow; to repair damaged tissue; to rebuild what has been worn down; and to renew their energies, as if you were planting them in the richest possible soil and helping them set roots and turn toward the sun.

Send that self back where they belong in your time line or find a refuge for them here by the stream.

Thank the helpers and your own compassionate self for the healing work you did here today.

If you want, you can just sit there and enjoy the space. Or, if you prefer, you can take a few moments to explore further along the pathway of this stream, into the stem if you have been in the cup, into the cup if you were down in the stem. Notice what condition this pathway is in. Where is it lush? Where are the surroundings sparse or unsupported? Where is it full or empty? Invite the Universal Supply Team in to help rehabilitate the pathway wherever it needs to be enriched and restored.

Now, place your hand again wherever you entered the stream and travel back to exit where you entered, if that is comfortable. Otherwise, choose your own exit point. Use your exhales to propel your awareness so that you feel your hand touching your body and your body being touched by that hand. Breathe in, exhale, breathe in, exhale. And open your eyes back to your everyday surroundings.

Know that you can return again and again, encounter your selves from different ages and dimensions, and console them.

Take a moment to jot down what you experienced.

☾ • ☽

The path of the next flow, the embodiment stream, always reminds me of those theater masks depicting joy and sorrow. It also makes me think of a line from a poem called "The Love Song of J. Alfred Prufrock" by T. S. Eliot: "There will be time, there will be time / To prepare a face to meet the faces that you meet."

Tracing Embodiment Stream (Stomach Meridian)

High Tide: 7 a.m. to 9 a.m.
Element: Earth
Direction: Yang
Trace this stream on both the left and right sides of your body.

Pull cosmic energy from the shared world to feed this stream as you trace it.

Place both hands beneath your eyes, on the tops of your cheekbones, in alignment with your pupils, one on each side of the midline. With your fingertips or palms, trace straight down to

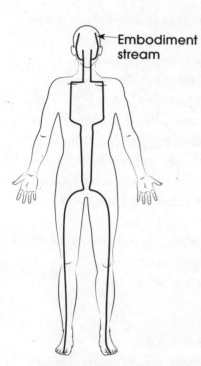

Embodiment stream

Figure 8.3. Embodiment stream (stomach meridian)

your jawbone and circle up the outside of your face to your forehead or hairline (see figure 8.3).

Then trace down over the centers of your eyes to your collarbones. Jog out at your collarbones.

Trace downward in a straight line.

Jog in at your waist, out at your hips, straight down the front of your legs, and off the second toes.

To clear or calm this stream, trace backward; to strengthen and support it, trace forward.

Guided Visit: Embodiment Stream

The cosmic feed for this stream comes from the shared world, our collective experience, and it enters via your eyes and mouth and face.

The embodiment stream helps you to stomach what comes at you, accept change, cope with the world, work with transitions, respond to events and energies of the world, embody your own truth, adapt your sense of yourself, and evolve as needed. It helps you "to prepare a face to meet the faces that you meet."

It is a good place to visit to explore digestion issues, both literal and figurative. It is also a good place in which to address challenges that affect your face, such as sinus congestion, and to work to calm sound sensitivity.

Embodiment energy is both strong and sensitive. It surrounds and embraces you, and when its flow is healthy, it can feel a bit protective or just warm and supportive.

Before you start, place your thumbs gently below each eye in line with your pupils, at the bottoms of your cheekbones, about level with the base of your nose. Place the rest of your fingers halfway up your forehead directly above each eye. Hold very lightly and gently. This hold helps to calm and balance your earth element.

Trace your embodiment stream from beneath your eyes, down to your jawline, up around the mask of the face, then down through your eyes and down your body off the second toe.

Get comfortable where you are sitting or lying down. Shut your eyes. Breathe in through your nose and out through your mouth. Feel and listen to your breath entering and leaving.

Now, find a place anywhere along the embodiment stream pathway to enter one side of the stream, either on the yin, or left, side of your body or on the yang, or right, side.

Shrink yourself down so you can travel along this pathway or just sink your attention down to enable you to explore and experience it.

What do you notice about your embodiment stream? Is it flowing gently or with some urgency? Is it active or sluggish, full or kind of empty? What else do your senses and mind pick up about this stream?

The cosmic roots of this flow come from the world, in through your face, midway between your eyes and mouth. What is coming through that entryway now? Imagine you turn to face a world you would like to inhabit, an ideal world. Imagine looking upon that world and, as you do that, notice if you feel any shifts in the energies of the stream.

Trace some metabolizing eights up and down the central part of this stream, from the base of your pelvis up to your eyes. How does this affect the stream? The feel of the energies?

Now, invite one of your selves (including from past lives) at a significant age, a self who needs to be accepted or healed or reformed, to join you here to receive support. Don't worry about which one to choose; you can always return here to meet with another one later. Invite guides or mentors to join you and help.

Ask this self what they need in order to accept themself and thrive; this is a place to give permission, acknowledgment, support. Ask yourself what conditions or expectations you need to let go of in order to accept this self.

As you interact with your alternate self, do a "Porcupine Reset" (pages 102–3) on them and/or on yourself to pull you both out of any kind of porcupine reactivity and to reinforce your gatekeeper's resilience. Figure-eight between you and that other self. Then trace (or help them trace on themselves) metabolizing eights along their center, to clear their sacred baton and bring in fresh nourishment. It is always lovely to do energy medicine when visiting one of the streams.

For those of you who can't easily accept, forgive, or support: ask that other self what they needed or lacked in their time and place. Invite guides to surround them and nourish and heal them over time. And offer them shelter somewhere along the stream. If for some reason that does not feel safe to do, then send them to a safe place off-site for now or back to their place on the time line, with a protector to accompany them.

Now, thank your former or future self for doing their best to embody your truth. Thank your present self for doing your best to let go of conditions and just accept. Thank the guides for helping you. And ask the stream what it needs from you in order to get healthier and to thrive. Stay open to how it wants to communicate. It might give you words, thoughts, an image, sounds, sensations, even a little movie scene.

When you are ready, place your thumbs again below each eye, at the base of your cheekbones, and your fingertips again halfway up your forehead, in line with your thumbs. Hold *very* lightly. Breathe in and exhale with whatever sound you want to make to help move the breath out. Now, place one hand on your heart and one hand on your solar plexus. Return your awareness first to your hands, breathing in and out, and then to the room around you. Open your eyes.

Take a moment to jot down anything you noticed about this stream.

◌ • ◌

GROUNDING IN HOW YOU KNOW

As you've seen, grounding is a rich spiritual practice of centering, release, anchoring, and rooting. By doing these, we become increasingly capable of accessing the inner guidance system built into each of us. We learn how to ground into our own wisdom and navigate via a true north signaled from within.

In these times of upheaval and change, a particularly important way we are being asked to evolve and ground is in *how* we know and hold our knowledge. With facts and other information easily at our fingertips via the internet, it is becoming increasingly crucial that we each learn to ground our minds into the core of our nature and our spiritual wisdom. It is important to make time to ground in the essence of our truth — our deepest values — and not just rely on things we read to tell us what is true. Without this practice, we can get caught in the illusion that opinion is fact or that a little information gleaned from unknown sources can substitute for lived experience and breadth of understanding.

Our language has many ways to express knowing: "I know it in my bones," "I know it in my heart," "I know it in my gut." As you evolve your ability to ground in a changing world, it is crucial to recognize these inner as well as outer ways of getting information and knowing. And it's important to learn how to validate your knowing in your body and spirit, as well as your socialized mind.

In chapter 9 we look at the issue of *coherence.* How can we hold body, mind, and soul together in the midst of change?

Chapter Nine

Holding Together
in the Face of Change

Irma ran a small business she had developed, and her husband chose the role of stay-at-home dad. Despite occasional lifted eyebrows and snide comments from neighbors, the marriage worked for them — until he was killed by a drunk driver. For the first six months, Irma held it all together, putting one foot in front of the other and getting on with what needed doing. But then she just lost it. She was a basket case, in a fog, unable to think, make decisions, or even take care of straightforward everyday tasks.

Martin and Helena worked hard to save the money to build their dream home in a small town where they intended to put down roots and raise their family. They were ready to start building when a tornado raged through the area and destroyed their town. Friends and family told them they were lucky that they hadn't lost everything, but they felt as though they had been punched in the gut and couldn't take a breath. Two years later, they were still on hold, unable to make decisions about how to move forward.

Angie was a triathlon athlete who spent much of her spare time training for various regional events. Early in 2020 she caught Covid-19 and spent three weeks feeling punky but congratulated herself on having a relatively mild case. Although she lost her sense of smell and taste and felt dizzy and tired, she was confident she would weather the virus just fine. But eight months later, when doctors assured her the virus was no longer in her system, she was still dizzy, tired, unable to smell or taste; she felt as though she had a slow leak somewhere that was draining her vitality and leaving her unable to work or play. She complained to friends that the virus had stolen her mojo.

What do these people have in common? They all went through an experience that wiped out the glue that held their energies together: their *coherence.*

When I think about the energetic concept of coherence, I often picture someone swinging a bucket full of water around and around themself. The water stays in the bucket as long as it keeps swinging, but if something stops the movement, the water splashes out, more often than not leaving them drenched and disoriented.

From a psychological perspective, you might say these people were processing shock, grief, and loss in the face of change. And this isn't incorrect. But there are *energetic* reasons why some people experience change and come out intact on the other side of the experience and some people lose their ability to function or thrive.

Your energies need to hold together, work in concert, stay woven, connected, and moving in sync. When you experience a big change, often your energetic glue gives way, and your energies lose their ability to communicate, coordinate, and work together.

Although the examples I gave above were negative experiences, you can also lose your energetic glue from a positive change.

When Ralph fell in love, he was in utter bliss for months. But he forgot to eat and sleep regularly and stopped seeing other friends while he and Jake were in their honeymoon period. And when they emerged, sharing a life together, Ralph was still sublimely happy. But he was exhausted. He couldn't catch up on sleep, and without sleep he couldn't focus on his day-to-day work. His naturopath diagnosed him with chronic fatigue syndrome. But that was the effect, not the cause. He, too, had wiped out his coherence, his energetic glue.

From a cosmic perspective, you are a swirling mass of energies. You are also a weave of strands of meaning formed as you experience and co-create your life with others. And in order for your moving, dancing strands of life force to work together, you need inner connection and coordination, you need your weave to hold its connections. Any change, shock, challenge, or transformation you go through can disrupt the weave. So it is extremely useful to know how to reinstate it. It is an important key to resilience within change and to healing long-term chronic illness or dysfunction.

What coherence do you need in order to thrive in the face of change?

- **You need coherence *within yourself*.** Your organs and anatomical and energetic systems need to work together. Medical testing sometimes misses the lack of coherence, since they don't have good tests to assess the ability of your parts to work in concert.
- **You need coherence *between parts of yourself*.** Not only do your body, mind, and spirit need to be in sync, but you also need congruence between the layers of yourself, between your inner identity and outer identity, between your selves at different ages. In other words, you need coherence in your various dimensions of self, so your gatekeeper knows which instructions to follow. Change almost always disrupts your identity in some way.
- **You need coherence *between your beliefs or thoughts and your actions*.** If your inner life doesn't match your lived experience or you are living a life that is not in keeping with your inner truth, this can degrade the glue that holds you together. Similarly, if you are pulled between your individual and group beliefs or needs, these too can damage your coherence.

FOUR DIMENSIONS OF ENERGETIC COHERENCE

My Councils have always encouraged me to "unpack" concepts, images, messages. They said, "Your minds [meaning all of us, not just me] are designed to perceive essences, shapes that embrace multiple meanings, and crossroads of meaning. If you unpack these, follow those roads, you will see where they lead and what the true significance of the crossroad is for you."

Here are four dimensions I like to work with when helping people cultivate better coherence:

- Connectors or energetic glue
- Purpose or guiding vision
- Structures or containers that unify your energies (explored in chapter 10)
- Integrations that get you in sync, creating congruence and alignment (also explored in chapter 10)

HOLDING TOGETHER

Connectors or *energetic glue* help to hold you together. Working with energetic connectors can be very healing to systems that don't work well because they aren't adequately linked.

I've already introduced a number of connectors in earlier pages of this book. Every time you do a hook-up hold to link two energy access points, for instance, you are providing glue. When you figure-eight between two points or trace a five-pointed star and circle over an area, you are connecting and integrating energies. When you use your interlaced fingers or do a Celtic weave (weaving your hands together in figure-eight motions) you also bring in coherence and connection.

Add in some of the everyday glue many of us have access to: shared laughter, pulling together with someone on a task (such as paddling a canoe), coordinating the details of a story, synchronizing your watches, or just getting a group on the same page with a unifying focus are all ways to bring energetic coherence.

But a particularly useful skill to learn is how to bring your own various parts into sync.

One morning when I was in my late teens, halfway between sleeping and waking, I had a dream that shimmered with significance. I think sometimes our Wiser Self sends us these dreams to alert us to something we need to understand or pay attention to. In the dream, I saw my body separating each night into layers, like those Russian nested dolls, and each layer went out into the world to have its own life and experiences. Then, right before waking, the individual layers would come running home and nest into my body, and I would wake up with the insights and knowing of each of those selves.

I wrote a poem about it, which has the distinction of being perhaps the worst poem I ever wrote. It was titled "My Body Is a Baklava"! What I saw in the dream was that each time my layers separated, the honey that should hold them together would dry out. My baklava layers could not stick together because I didn't have enough honey. In terms of my health, this was a form of inner and energetic burnout that has been a recurring challenge for me.

The energy body has layers to it, much like the baklava in my poem. When we are stressed, ungrounded, living a life that does not fully represent our truth, or subjected to some kind of gatekeeper challenge, the layers can lose their honey and come a bit unglued, causing energy drainage to the system and impeding intrabody communications. This can result in adrenal fatigue, discombobulation, or a sense of being foggy or fuzzy. It can also cause chrono-dysfunction — a challenge with orienting in time — and spatial disorientation as well. The following exercise, "Baklava Restoration," addresses these issues. It can be done by yourself or with a partner.

Exercise: Baklava Restoration

To Do This Exercise with a Partner

Stand approximately six feet behind your partner and put your palm at the level of their sacrum, facing their backside (see figure 9.1).

Ask your partner to imagine the layers of their baklava behind them. Have them breathe in and, on the exhale, slowly step back into the layers, gathering them together with each step. (This process might take several inhales and exhales.) Your hand will act as a bumper, unifying the layers of self and gluing them together at the sacrum.

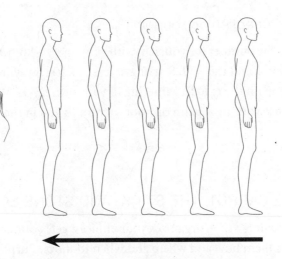

Figure 9.1. Baklava Restoration

Have your partner continue backing up on the exhale until their sacrum physically connects with your palm. Hold there for three to five seconds, to seal the layers together. You can also gently trace the five-pointed star and circle over the sacrum to help this correction hold (see figure 9.2).

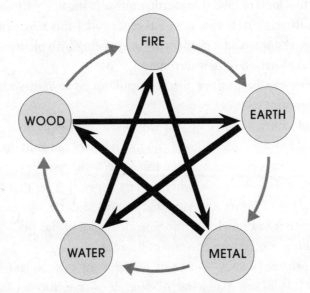

Figure 9.2. Tracing the five-pointed star and circle

To Do This Correction on Yourself

Use a wall as the bumper for yourself, with your energy-body layers standing between you and the wall. Starting at least six feet away from the wall, slowly back up on the exhale, gathering in your own layers. When you get to the wall, use your own palm on your sacrum to seal in the layers.

∽ • ∾

THE CARROT, THE STICK, AND STONE SOUP

Purpose or *guiding vision* organizes your choices, gets your energies moving, and tells them how and where and when to move. Purpose is like the harness that keeps horses trotting in tandem. It is also the destination that keeps you moving forward on your journey.

I am a little embarrassed to admit that I fall in love easily — with people, with ideas, with places, with new toys. I just revel in the sense of opening that happens when the wonder of one of these awakeners catalyzes me into exploration, new perspectives, or sheer pleasure in the awareness that this story or concept or amazing person is sharing the planet with me.

And that kind of love, that carrot, motivates me to sail through change gladly, embracing it. It tells my gatekeeper to let this new experience in and accept change. And it slathers my inner being with plenty of honey. It fuels the exploration of new territory.

Carrots can be positive teachers, pulling us toward situations our Wiser Self wants to experience.

But of course, as any of you who have overindulged in sugar also know, while a little honey is good, too much honey can gum up the works! There is a delicate balance between using carrots to provide coherence and tipping over into obsession, where I start depending on that new carrot to give me joy, or I start worrying that so-and-so doesn't love me back, or I discover that too much attention on this beloved has pulled my other relationships or commitments out of balance.

The proverbial stick — fear of punishment or loss, fear of missing out (FOMO), illness, pain, fear of disaster — can also act as energetic glue. Fear of global warming can push us to finally address our carbon footprint. Fear of getting sick can motivate us to take precautions and respect boundaries. Fear of reprisals can make me slow down and drive more sanely.

But for the most part, the stick can also break down your ability to move, choose, and act in holistic ways. It can wear down your body with stress hormones and your mind with defensive thinking. It can trigger your gatekeeper into reactivity when you least expect it. So sticks are mostly not great motivators.

If you find yourself hemmed in by fear or by people whose limitations limit you, then it is useful to cultivate your ability to identify *positive connectors*, purpose, and guiding vision that emanate from your core.

A stick can be transformed into a carrot if you are creative in finding the positive to emphasize even within tragedy. Remember Melanie and Jill, whose beloved forest burned down? They decided to use that stick as a carrot to guide their spiritual practice and deepen their understanding of nature.

Another way to create coherence in situations where you don't yet have the connectors you need is to use your *curiosity* as a stepping-stone.

Do you remember the children's story about stone soup? A stranger arrives in a village, hungry and tired. He has a cooking pot but no money to pay for food. The villagers eye him suspiciously, and he realizes they are not likely to open their hearts and share their food. So he fills his pot with water from the river, builds a fire where everyone can see him, puts his pot on to heat, and conspicuously drops in a stone drawn from his pocket.

Out of curiosity, the villagers edge closer. One asks, "What are you making?"

"Stone soup," he replies, "a most delicious delicacy."

A man asks, "Doesn't it have onions in it?"

"It could," says the traveler, "but I don't happen to have any with me."

The questioner volunteers a few onions. Another inquires about potatoes, with the same response. She drops a few potatoes into the pot. Then, one by one, the curious villagers contribute a bit of meat, some beans, other vegetables, spices. And the soup grows richer and more fragrant.

When the soup is ready, the visitor pockets his stone, and the villagers all share with him in the feast.

Curiosity and interest are, to my mind, some of the best glue. They are like the stone in stone soup, capable of pulling in resources, carrying us forward to outcomes we could not have controlled or produced on our own. They open us up to energetic exchanges we would not have otherwise experienced.

Because of our outside-in culture, we tend to think about purpose and goals in external terms. *What do I want my body to look like? How much money do I want to earn? How should I shape my career to get to where I want to go?*

But these external markers can just as easily destroy glue as create it. Consider the thirty-something lawyer pushing her body to exhaustion in her effort to achieve partner status. Consider the person who spends thousands of dollars on diets and coaching to look a certain way, only to wear down her metabolism in the process.

So this is another area where it is helpful to drop into your internal guidance system to find purpose and guiding vision from the inside out.

The two streams most fruitful for this, in my experience, sit in the element called wood in traditional Chinese medicine, which I think of as that aspect of living things that guides them to grow. Wood element has to do with taking the vital energy that comes to you and finding purpose and form to let your vision sprout from a seed and grow into a tree.

Tracing Purpose Stream (Liver Meridian)

High Tide: 1 a.m. to 3 a.m.
Element: Wood
Direction: Yin

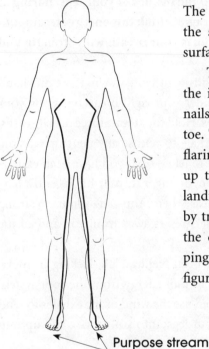

The cosmic source of this stream is the shared root systems below the surface of the earth.

To begin, place your fingers on the inside corners of your big toe-nails, between the big toe and second toe. Trace straight up inside the leg, flaring out at your hips, continuing up the front of your rib cage, and landing on your diaphragm. Finish by tracing along your diaphragm in the direction of the midline, stopping in line with your nipples (see figure 9.3).

Purpose stream

Figure 9.3. Purpose stream
(liver meridian)

Guided Visit: Purpose Stream

Reach down into the shared root system beneath the earth to find the cosmic source of this stream.

Your purpose flow is a place to come when you need to support growth or address overgrowth of cells, thoughts, or behaviors in your body, mind, or spirit. It is a place to come to find your strength and your flexibility, your courage of conviction. It is also a place to transform anger into purpose or frustration into a path forward. It is a place to come to support vision, both literal and figurative.

Trace both sides of your purpose flow, reaching first into the cosmic source within the mycelium and root systems of the earth, then tracing from inside your big toe, up the insides of your legs, flaring at the hips, and ending on your diaphragm. Hook this energy stream into the diaphragm muscle, which supports your breath with strength and purpose.

Get comfortable where you are sitting or lying down. Place one hand on your high heart and the other under your right breast, covering your liver and right rib cage. Shut your eyes. Hold for at least three deep breaths.

Breathe in and out, using the exhale to release any pent-up tension, emotions, or stale energies you want to let go of. If you have been experiencing logjammed energy, frustration, or anger in your life recently, harness the winds of your exhales to release them. You can even use a strong puffing sound or shout to send these stresses away from you and all the way out of your energy field.

If, on the other hand, you have been feeling blah, lacking in motivation or strength, use your inhales to pull energy from the root system under the earth into your feet and then use the wind of the exhales to send that root energy upward through your legs, into your torso, and up into your head, bathing your eyes with it.

Now, shrink down to enter your purpose flow at any point along its pathway, on either side of your body, or sink your attention down into the stream.

What do you notice there? Use all your senses to pick up what you feel, hear, see, think, smell, and taste in this place. What is the energy of this stream? Is it moving or still? Clear or polluted? Full or empty? Just notice its qualities and commune with wherever you find yourself.

What is growing in this place? Are there trees or other plants around? What is the landscape this stream is flowing through, as you perceive it?

If you can, find a tree growing here that you can explore. If you see no trees around, invite one into this space. Trees live in the three realms: within the earth, upon the earth, and in the sky. The roots dive into invisible depths with incredible outreach. The trunk brings strength and conducts water and nutrients from the roots to the branches and leaves, which give the tree flexibility to blow with the wind.

If you are comfortable doing so, enter the tree or become one with it, or just embrace it or lean against it. Feel it spanning the three worlds. Send your awareness down into the root system to explore what you feel or perceive there; this is a wonderful place to go to get to know your connectedness with all life-forms. If you wish, while sitting within its roots, ask a question of the tree and note what arises in your mind and inner vision.

Now, travel upward into the tree to become its trunk. Notice what that feels like for you. Can you feel water or nutrients traveling through you as you meld with or inhabit this form? If you wish, you can pose a question to the tree — or to yourself — about how you can evolve or move forward in embodying well-being.

Now, travel further upward, into the canopy of the tree. What season is it? Are there leaves or nuts, blossoms or fruits, or perhaps just bare branches? What is the wind like? How does it feel to be one with this canopy, moving with the wind?

This is a place where transformation is a constant. Feel the cycle of life the tree goes through season by season, the magic of converting sunlight to carbohydrates that feed the tree and nourish its many changes. If you wish to ask for insights of the tree here, this is a wonderful place to brainstorm or plan.

When you are ready, bring your consciousness back down into the trunk of the tree and then into the trunk of your body and breathe. Separate yourself from the tree, recognizing both the connections you have made and your separate nature.

Return your attention to the flow of purpose that lives in this place. How clear or pure is this energy now? How is it polluted, backed up, or otherwise compromised? Call on the Universal Supply Team to come in to filter, cleanse, and purify the stream, as needed.

If you wish, scoop up some of the energies from the stream and bring them to your eyes. Cup your hands over your eyes and infuse your whole visual apparatus with healing energies, including the parts of your brain that support vision.

Now, thank the stream and your tree for whatever you have learned here today. Ask the tree for seeds you can take with you. Keep them to plant later in the enactor/enforcer stream, which is the yang partner of the purpose stream. Place your hands again on your body, one on the high heart, the other over your liver below your right breast.

Breathe in through your nose and out through your mouth, feeling the breath as a kind of wind that enlivens your body. Feel it entering, spreading, and exiting and feel the pause as you are empty. And notice the moment it begins the new cycle, entering your nose. Watch your breath through one more cycle and then open your eyes, bringing your attention to the room you are in.

Take a moment to jot down what you experienced.

∞ • ∞

CONFLICTS AND DOUBLE BINDS

When two horses hitched to a carriage pull together in the same direction, the carriage moves forward. When they pull in opposite directions, the carriage spins — and often ends up upside down in a ditch!

One of the best ways to wipe out your energetic glue is to get caught in conflicts and double binds. Pulling yourself in many different directions or working at cross-purposes with other members of your family or circle can drain your energies quickly and effectively. This does not mean you always have to go along with what others want. But the ability to find the larger mind understandings that pull you out of binary struggles becomes a crucial energy support.

When you find yourself in a double bind — damned if you do and damned if you don't — try plugging your concerns into the stabilizing sphere (pages 88–92) or else enter the enactor/enforcer stream to activate your ability to move forward and grow beyond the present snag.

Tracing Enactor/Enforcer Stream (Gallbladder Meridian)

High Tide: 11 p.m. to 1 a.m.
Element: Wood
Direction: Yang
Trace this stream on both the left and right sides of your body.

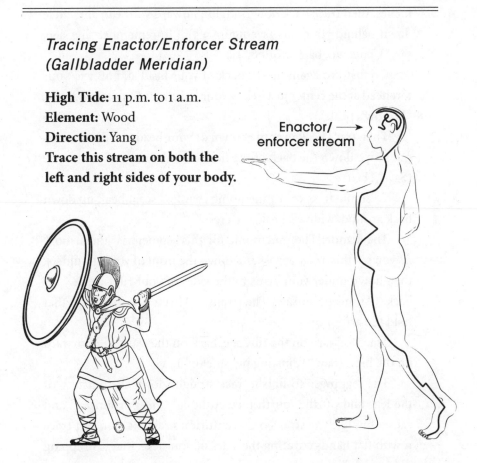

Figure 9.4. Roman centurion

Figure 9.5. Enactor/enforcer stream (gallbladder meridian)

This flow is easier to remember if you picture a Roman centurion, steadfast and loyal, wearing his gear! (See figure 9.4.)

Access to the cosmic flow of this stream comes through donning the helmet of service.

The helmet: Place the fingers of each hand on the outer edges of your eyebrows, both sides at once.

Trace with your fingers from your eyebrows to the openings of your ears. (As a mnemonic, repeat the oath "I see, I hear.")

Now trace straight upward with your fingertips about two

inches, then trace back down, angling toward your ear, and circle down behind your ears (see figure 9.5). (To remember this step, say, "Up, down, back around.")

Go forward again up the back of your head and over to your forehead at the center just below your hairline. (To remember, say, "Widow's peak.")

Then trace back over the crown of your head and draw a central stripe down the back of the helmet to the nape of your neck. (Say, "The crest.")

To summarize your mnemonic chant: "I see, I hear, up down back around, widow's peak, the crest."

The armor: The mnemonic for this segment is "the armor." As you say this, trace across and down the front of your shoulders, then down under your arms to the sides of your rib cage at your back. (At this point say, "The straps.") This is like the straps that hold the armor on.

Trace forward on the rib cage, back on the waist, and forward on the hips. (Say, "Adjusting my shields.")

The leggings: To finish, trace straight down the outsides of the legs and off the fourth toes. Although this portion zigs and zags a bit, like the straps on a centurion's sandals, you can trace it with flat hands covering the sides of your legs. (Say, "Strapping my sandals.")

Note: the fourth finger of the hand is the start of your energizer flow (Triple Warmer). This enactor/enforcer flow comes off the fourth toe: it is like a lieutenant that enacts and enforces the decisions of the general, your energizer flow.

Guided Visit: Enactor/Enforcer Stream

Access to the cosmic source comes through donning the helmet of service.

This stream is a good place to find your willingness to live your truth, to serve your truth. It is also a good place to let go of any feelings you might be

holding on to: anger, resentment, emotions about past experiences, restless-
ness — everything that doesn't serve that truth in this moment.

This enactor/enforcer stream contains the energy that activates the un-
folding of seeds: literal seeds and seed ideas, new paths, and new choices. If
there are any decisions you are trying to make in your life, or conflicts, double
binds, or problems you are trying to resolve, let the spirits of this place speak
to you. Ask for clarity, guidance, and practical suggestions.

Trace your enactor/enforcer flow on both sides of your body, break-
ing the process down into three parts: the helmet, the armor, and the
leggings. As you trace, call in the cosmic energy of service.

Get comfortable where you are lying or sitting down. Close your eyes
and place your hands on the sides of your head, as though holding your
helmet. Breathe in through your nose and out through your mouth, then
again in through your nose and out through your mouth.

As you inhale, breathe in willingness to live your truth, to serve your
truth. Exhale and let go of any feelings or thoughts you might be holding
on to: anger, resentment, memories of past experiences, restlessness. Release everything that doesn't serve your truth in this moment.

Now, place your hands on the sides of your rib cage, as if holding your
body armor. And again breathe in through your nose, out through your
mouth. As you inhale, feel your strength of purpose. As you exhale, let go
of anything that pulls you away from your purpose. Feel each in and out
breath building your strength to fulfill your potential, to support your
healthiest evolution and growth.

Now, place your hands on the sides and backs of your knees, holding
there lightly as you breathe in through your nose and out through your
mouth. Breathe in a sense of purpose and, as you exhale, feel yourself
ready to step up and act, as needed, to embody your soul's truth and support your gatekeeper in protecting your being.

Choose any point to enter your enactor/enforcer stream on the left
or right side of your body. Shrink down or sink your attention down into
the stream. Explore what you find here. What do you perceive about this
energy flow and the space that it inhabits?

What is the strength of this flow? How full is the stream? Is its path
straight or meandering? What is growing here, and how would you assess

the ecology of this place? Balanced? Out of balance? How do you feel as you visit this stream?

If there are plants, are they growing well or overgrown, in need of some pruning? Are they thriving or needing to be tended? Call upon a master gardener to come in and care for the plant life here, to bring this space into balance and harmony, to help it fulfill its potential.

Ask the master gardener if there is a master plan or design. Will they show it to you or tell you something about it? Ask them what you can do to support the plan and/or the health of this place.

Now, also ask where you should go to plant the seeds you gathered from your visit to your purpose flow. The right spot may well be somewhere along this stream. But stay open — the master gardener might surprise you by suggesting a totally different place to plant those seeds. Follow their suggestions as best you can and plant the seeds. If it is not a place you can get to, you can give the seeds to the master gardener to plant on your behalf.

As you plant the seeds or hand them over for planting, bless them and ask for help converting your intentions to action. Dip a cup into the stream to water your planted seeds with the energy of activation. If you wish, you can drink from the stream or dip into it in any way you feel comfortable.

Now, sit for a spell beside the flow and just notice your surroundings. If you feel called to explore other areas of the stream — the area around the armor or leggings if you are up in the helmet, the leggings or helmet if you are in the armor — go ahead and do so. If you are struggling to resolve problems or conflicts or to free yourself from ways you feel trapped or stuck, ask the spirits of this place to give you guidance and practical suggestions.

Note what comes up for you, what your attention is drawn to. And notice whether you find yourself judging the situation or what is arising in your mind. If so, breathe in and let the judgments go with your exhale. Know that just as you don't need to tell a plant how to grow, you don't need to push for answers. They will be given form and delivered to you when the time is right.

Thank the master gardener and the spirits of this place for their help and service. And once again hold the sides of your helmet, then the sides of your armor, then hold lightly behind your knees. Breathe in through your nose and out through your mouth, feeling your hands touching your body and your body being touched. Bring your awareness to your body, sitting or lying here, and open your eyes.

Take a moment to jot down what you experienced.

∽ • ∽

The more you work with purpose and let it inform your actions, the more honey you will generate to hold your baklava together from within. Coherence is also supported by inner and outer structure, by strengthening the weave of your fabric, as we will explore in chapter 10.

∽ Chapter Ten ∾

Reweaving the Tears
in Your Fabric

Breathing is one of nature's best ways to restore your coherence. That is probably why it is integral to most spiritual and healing practices. Your breath:

- carries in and delivers life-giving oxygen
- activates the binaries and cycles that run your body
- supports your nervous system in both windup and release
- fuels your brain
- sets a tempo for all your physical processes
- acts as a connecting thread

It gives structure, and it weaves your energies together — breath is excellent energy medicine! Whenever you are befuddled by change or wishing to fuel a transformation, it is helpful to make time to return to your breath and tune in to its journey.

Your body has several built-in metronomes that set a beat to coordinate all of your energies to work together. Your heart sets the beat for the circulation of your energies and fluids; your elemental rhythm sets the tempo for how you can most productively move; and your breath supports the through line of your song, your everyday actions.

Consider for a moment which tempo best suits you in your truest form:

- **Water element** moves in a *slow and stately* way but is comfortable when *still and deep* or can *rush when pressed.*
- **Wood element** moves *briskly,* pushing through obstacles with purpose and in a *clear, linear* manner, like the plant pushing through soil and upward to reach the sunlight.
- **Fire element** *dances and leaps* from place to place while also *lighting the way* and *warming* those around it.
- **Earth element** evolves with time, moving in a *rolling rhythm,* meandering to cover more ground, but generally *progressing forward.*
- **Metal element** moves with *efficient dignity,* generally cutting through obstructions and taking the *shortest, most direct route,* with clarity of understanding in how to get where it needs to go.

If you are an earthy soul but are expected to produce your work at a rapid clip, that can destroy your coherence and dysregulate your body's rhythms.

Similarly, if you are a woody soul but are asked to bide your time and work slowly, it can send your systems into overdrive, also pulling your energies out of sync.

Your personal ability to keep your glue fresh and vital depends in part on your elemental makeup; it is bound up in the pace with which you live. It is also bound up in the structures and containers that frame your experience.

Sami was a refugee who lost her home, undergoing a horrendous journey through hostile territory and a couple of different refugee camps before she found her way to Canada. It was a traumatizing experience for her, but she was pragmatic and determined to just keep moving forward and adapt.

Back home, she had been a family-law advocate. She had to reinvent herself when she arrived in her new home, because she wasn't licensed and didn't yet have enough English to work in any real professional capacity.

Although she was determined to be present and stay in the here and now, she had trouble sleeping, then started experiencing anxiety attacks. From there, she developed irritable bowel syndrome (IBS) but dismissed it by telling herself she was just reacting to stress. She ignored all these symptoms until she began to experience pain and bruising all over her body.

When she consulted a doctor, he diagnosed a connective tissue disorder. In fact, he told her that her body was disintegrating. He said, "There's no cure. Maybe we can give you some drugs to slow it down, but it is a degenerative disease, and you probably can only live a few more years."

She sought out energy medicine help because she did not accept his death sentence. Of course, she needed to work to calm her gatekeeper, needed to reground her energies in this new land, but most of all, she needed to address coherence: how to bring integration to her dis-integrating body.

When someone like Sami loses the structures in their life — she lost her language, most of her family, her grounding in her home territory, her profession, and the shared history with her community — their gatekeeper can lose its identity, and their body and mind can come apart at the seams.

Sami was extremely pragmatic. She just determined to assimilate into Canadian society and move ahead with efficient dignity. (Can you tell her dominant elemental rhythm was metal?) But her body did not get the memo. It lacked the structures it needed, and she had not taken the time to reweave the tears in her fabric. Without coherence, her body's connective tissue began to disintegrate.

Part of what she needed was to reclaim what she could: to speak her mother tongue, to meet with others from her country, to honor her grief and loss and filaments of connection that had been ripped asunder. And she also needed to work to find new coherence: new structures to support her and meaningful new patterns of activity that would reweave her energies from the inside out.

When she did this, her body miraculously recovered from the supposedly incurable disease.

WHAT SUPPORTS YOU

Structures or containers that unify your energies are important. We need context that links our individual choices to a larger identity and meaning.

Energetic containers are more than just boxes and Tupperware. They include any unifying factors that provide structure or contain your energies, thereby bringing coherence. In the exploration below, you'll recognize a number of tools from earlier chapters.

ᥩ Play with It! ᥩ

1. **Framing:** Place the area of concern into some kind of frame or container. This can be a conceptual or physical framework or else an energetic one.

   If you have an organ or part of your life that isn't working, try using your hands to trace an energetic shape or frame around the organ or situation. Or experiment with drawing a large seedpod around your whole body. This will contain your body's energies and your aura in a protective shell.

2. **Unifying focus:** Use something that focuses your energy, like a mantra.

   Try singing a scale or counting from one to ten while breathing slowly in and out.

3. **Rhythm:** Find a rhythm that acts like an orchestra conductor to get your energies synced to the same beat.

   Place one hand over a part of your body that feels discombobulated; with your other hand, tap a rhythm on the hand holding the body.

   You can relieve tired eyes by placing one finger across a closed eyelid, then tapping that finger to a rhythm.

4. **Energy overlay:** Flood the area with a stronger energy to help it organize.

Trace hearts or figure eights all over your body (or the situation you want to bring more coherence to). Or bathe yourself in color. Or surround yourself with music that creates unity for you.

5. **Pace:** Like setting a beat, change the pace to focus the energies so they can work more coherently together.

Go for a brisk or meandering walk. Take a day of rest. Entrain your energies to someone who is coherent.

6. **Story line / plot:** Identify a plot or story line for what is happening; it should link events into a framework that makes sense of them and relieves stress.

Try telling a story that explains your uncomfortable events. For example, when a driver cuts me off on the freeway, nearly causing an accident and making my gatekeeper explode with rage, I offer myself a fictional explanation: "He's rushing to the hospital to be there for his wife's surgery." That story releases my compassion, and then I can send him good wishes to get there safely and on time.

7. **Vision, intention, plan, goal:** Goals can paint you into a corner, but they can also stimulate your energies in good ways.

Instead of setting a goal to change yourself (lose weight, get in shape, put yourself out there professionally), set some exploration or project for yourself that is motivated by curiosity and pleasure. For example, decide that for one day you are going to seek out as many nonfood things that nourish you as you can; you'll eat only foods that bring you strong pleasure; and you will take only as many bites as provide that pleasure.

8. **Weaves and webworks:** Link your actions, choices, and events into a larger structure.

Try the "Zigzag Hook-Up" (pages 157–59) to weave together your core energies. Tell a story that connects your struggle to a larger social movement or family pattern.

∽ • ∾

INNER STRUCTURE

Integrations: congruence, alignment, getting in sync strengthen inner structure. It is common to think of structure as a kind of scaffolding that holds everything in place and gives it shape, like your skeleton. But because our energies are a moving dance, how that dance moves and coordinates within itself is another aspect of inner structure. Working on bringing your energies into a healthier sync strengthens your resilience and ability to thrive.

Our energies form a matrix of moving exchanges that emanate from a deep grid your soul lays down as an interface between your source and your body. Stress, grief, loss, shock, and radical change can put pressure on this grid, torquing its weave, snapping its threads, and leaving you feeling utterly untethered inside.

Sami lost more than the outer trappings of her former life when she had to leave her homeland. She came unraveled inside. But she was able to use the "Body Weave" protocol below to support her deepest warp and weft.

Protocol: Body Weave

1. Starting at the base of your left pelvis and at your left collarbone (see the two points labeled 1 in figure 10.1), hold your hands flat (or use fingertips if that is more comfortable) at the top and bottom to reinforce your first vertical warp line. Hold until you take a deep breath or feel these lines click into place and achieve a good tension (see figure 10.2).

    If the line between these two points does not feel solid, you can reinforce it with color or sound until you feel it has got a good, solid feel to it. Use whatever color feels right.

    If this warp line feels like a clogged tube and needs clearing, blow sharply into the top as you would to clear a drinking straw or tube.

2. Then move to the next points on your pelvic floor and collarbone (points 2, second in from your left side) and hold until you feel this vertical line clicks in or you take a deep breath.

Adjust with color or sound and use breath to clear if needed.

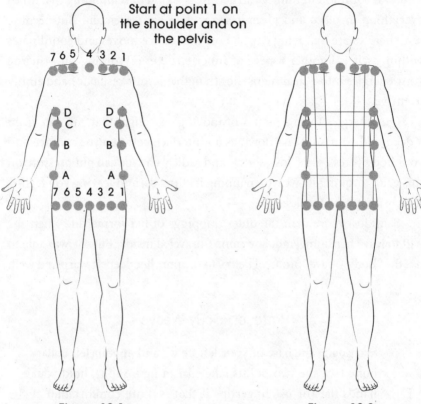

Figure 10.1.
Body Weave points

Figure 10.2.
Vertical and horizontal weave

3. Proceed to hold and reinforce lines 3 through 7 in the same manner, until you feel you have a solid warp to weave on.

4. Now it is time to weave your horizontal weft lines. Starting at the A point on your left side (see figure 10.1), move your hand in a waving in-and-out motion along your pelvic floor, as if you are weaving a horizontal thread over the first warp line, under the second, over the third, and so on. Continue until you have woven all the way to the A point on your right side (see figure 10.2). Then hold the A points on the side of each

hip, both at the same time, until you feel this horizontal weft settle in and feel solid.

5. Continue to the B points at your waist. First use the weaving motion from left to right across your torso, then hold both sides of your waist until you feel the weft line settle in and hook up.

6. Proceed to the C points at your rib cage. Again make the weaving motion from left to right with your hand, then hold both sides of your ribs until you feel the weft line settle in and hook up.

7. Next, weave in the same manner between your D points, then hold and connect your D points at your armpits. You can hold with your thumbs tucked in your armpits and fingers covering the front of your shoulder, where your arm attaches to your body. Or cross your arms for this hold, if that is easier.

8. Finish by tracing a figure eight on each of the diagonals, from left hip to right shoulder and from right hip to left shoulder. Then hold both hands on your heart and breathe love and radiance into your renewed weave.

∽ • ∾

Because Sami was disintegrating inside herself rather than outwardly, in her everyday life, she was able to get valuable ongoing guidance from her body by entering the two metal element streams: the give and receive flow and the distiller/refiner flow. Metal element supports structure and the expression of spirit into form, so they were perfect places for her to hang out and let her body show her the way.

Tracing Give and Receive Stream (Lung Meridian)

High Tide: 3 a.m. to 5 a.m.
Element: Metal
Direction: Yin

Give
and
receive
stream

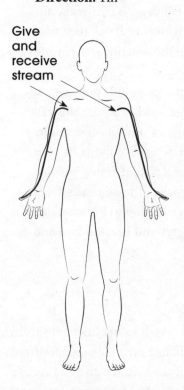

Pull loving cosmic energy from the heart of the world to fill your hands prior to tracing this stream.

To trace the flow, place one hand over the opposite lung and trace up to the front of your shoulder, straight down your arm in line with your thumb, and off your thumb (see figure 10.3).

When that is complete, switch hands and trace the other side.

To strengthen this flow, trace it forward, as described above. To clear or calm the flow, trace it backward from thumb to lung.

Figure 10.3. Give and receive
stream (lung meridian)

Guided Visit: Give and Receive Stream

The cosmic source for this stream comes into you by way of your heart chakra, which spirals out and pulls enrichment in from the world.

This stream is a place to come to give and receive awareness, resources, faith, breath, or the life force that your spirit and body and mind need in order to be truly alive. It is also a place to let go of whatever does not serve you.

It's a good stream to visit if you have lung or breathing issues.

Trace the path of this stream on each side of your body, starting at your lung and pulling the energy down your arm, off your thumb. Extend the pull of energy out to arm's length, to support better release.

Get comfortable where you are lying or sitting down. (This visit is especially good to do lying down.) Close your eyes and tune in to your breath. Without trying to control it, notice what your breath is doing. Pay attention to the moment it begins to enter your nostrils, notice the lift of your chest, feel what happens to your lower belly and diaphragm as you inhale.

And notice the moment when you begin to exhale. What happens to your belly, diaphragm, chest, and nostrils as you exhale? What do you feel as you breathe in and out? What do you hear? Or smell?

Allow the rhythm of your breath to fill your awareness. You *are* your nose, and the pathways for the air, and the apparatus of breathing. Let them breathe, and just observe.

Experiment with breathing in through your nose and out through your mouth. How does that change the breathing?

Place one hand on your heart chakra, at the center of your chest, and the other on your solar plexus. Notice how that affects your breathing.

Allow the hand on your heart chakra to absorb cosmic energy until you feel the hand is saturated with it. Then reach that hand across to the lung on the opposite side of your body and cover your lung with your hand, allowing the cosmic energies to filter in with the inhale.

Shrink yourself down or sink your attention down into the give and receive stream at any point you feel drawn to enter. What do you notice about this stream, using all of your senses? What do you hear, feel, see, taste, smell, or know in this place?

Explore the stream. How strong is its flow? How clean or polluted is this stream and the place it flows through? Invite the Universal Supply Team in to clean up all that obstructs or pollutes this place and to restore it to its most pristine natural, healthy state.

Next, invite guides in to join you. Ask your guides, "What do I need in order to be well?" Ask them, "Where should I send the energies that do not serve me?"

Now, find somewhere along this stream where you can comfortably lie down on the earth, at least in your mind's eye. Allow your weight to sink down into the ground and feel the ground holding you. Let your body take over the breathing and give yourself over to the earth, which is supporting you. And then, if you can, let the earth itself take over and breathe you. Like a baby lying on its mother's chest, feel the rise and fall, the breath within mother earth, breathing you. Feel yourself in utter sync with the breath of the mother, held and warm in her embrace. Let your mind sink into the pure sensations of being breathed by the loving being that holds you.

When you are ready, thank the mother for giving you the breath of life.

Slowly, bring your attention back into your own breathing apparatus, still feeling the giving and receiving rhythms of the earth. Now notice your individual breaths entering, resting, leaving, and resting empty.

Spread your arms out to receive blessings from the heavens, fill your hands with those blessings, and bring both hands to your heart or lungs, to feed them with heaven's bounty.

Leaving both hands on your chest, breathe in through your nose and out through your mouth. Feel the warmth of your hands and the rise and fall of your chest or belly as you breathe. When you are ready, find a place to exit the stream and bring your attention fully back to your body, whether you are sitting or lying down. And slowly move around to return to your everyday consciousness. Open your eyes.

Take a moment to jot down what you experienced.

☙ • ❧

Tracing Distiller/Refiner Stream (Large Intestine Meridian)

High Tide: 5 a.m. to 7 a.m.
Element: Metal
Direction: Yang

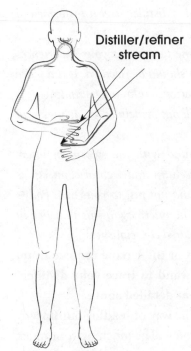

Distiller/refiner stream

Figure 10.4. Distiller/ refiner stream (large intestine meridian)

Access the cosmic source of the distiller/refiner stream via your index (pointer) finger. Plug it into the heart of the Divine for a Divine hook-up.

Placing the open fingers of one hand at the end of the pointer finger of the opposite hand, trace straight up the back of your arm, from the fingertip, to your shoulder (see figure 10.4). Continue inward along your collarbone to your neck, then up the side of your neck. From there trace to the base of your nose and cross under your nose, ending at the flare of your nose on the opposite side.

Switch hands and repeat on the second side.

Notice that the two sides of distiller/refiner flow cross over each other and cradle your nose, influencing not only your sense of smell but also your brain.

Guided Visit: Distiller/Refiner Stream

Access the cosmic source for the distiller/refiner flow via your index (pointer) finger. Plug it into the heart of the Divine for a Divine hook-up.

Your head, your heart, and your gut form three brains that work together to keep your energies moving and coherent. Your gut separates the food and energies you have digested into nutrients and refuse. It releases what your body cannot use and creates over thirty energetic messengers, neurotransmitters that regulate the workings of your head and heart and body. It is the place where what you take in from the world is distilled and transformed to serve your body, mind, and spirit.

This stream is a wonderful place to come to sort out your experiences and understand what you can use and what should be released. It is a place to come to transform painful or positive experience into understanding. It is a place to visit to learn lessons and then distill out principles, guidelines, and concepts to inform your future choices.

This energetic stream is intimately bound with the swarm of interconnections, with the root systems and mycelium and web of connections that link all of creation. The cells here respond not just to your own body's needs but to the collective consciousness of the microorganisms that live in your gut and in the earth, as well as to the shared consciousness.

Plug your index finger into the heart of the Divine to juice it up. Then use your index finger as a magic wand to trace your distiller/refiner stream on each side of your body, as detailed above.

We are going to use a mudra, a symbolic way of holding our fingers, in this visit. With the pad of your thumb, you will be touching your index finger at the base of the nail on the side facing your thumb. Practice that mudra now.

Get comfortable where you are sitting or lying down and close your eyes. Place each hand flat at the base of your torso, cradling your large intestine and gut-brain area. If possible, while still cradling your gut, make the mudra described above with your thumb and index finger of each hand. Breathe in through your nose and out through your mouth.

Continue to breathe in through your nose and out through your mouth, using your exhales to release any tension or energy or feelings or thoughts you want to let go of. In through your nose, out through your mouth...feel free to moan and groan to support the release.

Now, release your mudras, and if it is comfortable for you to do so, leave your right hand cradling your gut while you reach out with your left index finger to plug into the heart of the Divine. If your arms aren't comfortable doing this, you can invite the Divine to come to you, to link with your index finger wherever it is comfortable.

Send the Divine energy coming into your left index finger out through your right hand into your gut. Hold this Divine hook-up until you feel your gut responding, receiving the Divine energy. Then, continuing the Divine hook-up, move your right hand across to the left side of your gut and bring Divine energy there as well.

Now, find a place where you feel drawn to enter your left or right distiller/refiner pathway. Place your hand at that spot and shrink yourself down or sink your attention down to enter the stream.

Using all of your senses, including your thoughts, what do you notice about this place? What does the flow feel like to you? Is there movement, or is it still? Is the flow clear, or are there obstructions? Does the stream seem healthy, or does it need some support from the Universal Supply Team? If it needs support, call them in now and ask them to help you rehabilitate and revitalize this stream. Allow them to help you and invite them to show you what you can do to help them.

Is there something in your health, emotions, or life you would like to understand better? You have two choices here. If it is a puzzling but not painful situation, you can look around for a comfortable spot to settle near the stream and invite in clarity and insight. Anchor yourself in the stabilizing sphere and just let this place work to clarify your energies.

If your situation is painful, agonizing, or causing you grief, look around for a dark cave, a grotto, a place where you can be separate and alone and sit in darkness. Enter that dark place. Focus on what is most challenging and/or painful about your situation. Where are you feeling that focus? Is it a thought in your brain, a feeling in your heart, or a sensation in your gut? Experiment with moving the challenge to each of these three brains in turn. Hold it with compassion and love; if there is pain or sorrow, breathe into it. Don't try to change it for now. Simply try to meet it and recognize it and acknowledge it.

Ask the challenge what it wants you to know. You are not trying to solve problems in this moment, but rather just meeting this challenge intimately, in your head, heart, and gut. If it is painful, just keep breathing into the pain. Ask yourself if you can stand to accept the pain for the space of three deep breaths. If the answer is yes, breathe and sit with the pain or challenge as is.

Notice as you breathe if anything is shifting. If not, see if you are willing to sign on to sit with the challenge for three more long breaths. Again, just sit with the challenge or pain, not trying to change it, and notice if it starts to transform on its own. If not, keep breathing and accepting, until you feel light entering this space or you feel you need to emerge from the darkness to a lighter place for now.

The cells in this place respond not just to your own body's needs but to the needs of the microorganisms that live in your gut and in the earth and to the shared consciousness. Ask the swarm of microorganisms in the earth to send you healing energies and resources to help you on your path.

Feel your body sending roots from every pore of your skin, every cell of your body, down into the ground to receive that help. Call upon whatever you hold sacred — Goddess or God, love of animals, truth — to sanctify and tune this help to a frequency that supports your Earth Elemental Self to thrive as a unity. If you wish, you can sing a consoling note or bathe in a unifying color or draw a supportive shape upon or around your body. Or put your body into an energetic seedpod for protection.

Breathe in through your nose and out through your mouth. Although this stream is a yang flow, a releaser, it provides important information to your yin gatekeeper, via the vagus nerve. Invoke again whatever you feel reverent about, whatever stirs your spirit. Infuse the entire stream with that energy and ask the web of consciousness of microorganisms to resonate and amplify that energy as well. Send it up through your vagus nerve to infuse your heart and head with this truth.

Thank the spirits of the place, and the Universal Supply Team, and your own tender heart and gut and brain, and place both hands over your gut again, cradling it. Find a place to exit the stream and return your consciousness to the surface. Breathe in and out, bringing your attention to your hands touching your skin and your skin being cradled by your hands. And when you are ready, open your eyes to the present moment.

Jot down whatever you learned or experienced in your visit to this stream.

◌ • ◌

In our everyday language, we have lots of ways to say we are lacking coherence: "I can't hold it together," "I'm coming apart at the seams," "I'm feeling all torn up," "I am at sixes and sevens," "I'm falling apart," "I'm discombobulated," "I'm all to pieces," "I've lost the thread," and more. We all understand coherence — and its lack — experientially. Energy medicine gives you the tools to pull your energies together, shift your weave, and support your deepest fabric to hold strong.

∞ Chapter Eleven ∞

Flow

When I encounter change, sometimes it makes me stop, roll up into a tight ball like a pill bug, and wait for the world to stop spinning. And sometimes, it sends me into overdrive, so I'm flooded with plans, ideas, enthusiasm, and to-do lists. Mostly, I tend to hop in with both feet, then freak out afterward, when I realize what I've taken on.

You might recognize that these are gatekeeper reactions. But they are also ways that life influences the *flow* of the moving, swirling mass of energies that I'm made of.

In the art form that is *navigating change*, working with the flow of your energies can make the difference between health and illness, enjoying change or suffering it, recovering from the unexpected or having it deepen into trauma.

When you think about it, movement is life. If your brain or heart or lungs stop their activity, you are dead. If your circulation is impeded or insufficiently pumped, organs and body parts falter. If your brain is clogged, or sluggish, or stuck in a closed loop, it doesn't work as efficiently. And if you stay still for too long, your body signals its discontent with aches and pains that usually release once you restore circulation and movement.

Think about trying to steer a car. If the car is at a standstill, it is extremely difficult to turn the steering wheel. But when you gently set the car in motion, the wheel turns easily, and you can have a say in where that car is going. When your car is traveling at safe speeds for the road conditions, a small turn of the wheel can have a big impact.

Just as too little movement is problematic, so is overactivity. Overexercising can wear your body down. If you try to turn when speeding faster than conditions warrant, you will find your car careening off the road. And too much movement can flood rather than support your flows, causing your subtle energies to miss their mark and fail to nourish you.

Your subtle energies need to move, and they need space to get where they are going. That's one reason that movement, stretching, and gesture are great forms of energy medicine.

But your subtle energies also need to move at a pace and rhythm that is right for your body and nature: they need to flow the way they are designed to flow, in certain patterns. Otherwise, like with a river, you can run into dry riverbeds, flooding, pollutants from energies not meant to be there, and stress for the life-forms that make up the ecology of each stream.

When change disrupts your movement, rhythm, pace, direction, patterns, or ability to steer, then knowing how to consciously work with these to influence the flow of your subtle energies and of your life becomes a gift and a necessity. Working with flow is a key to healing both your body and your life!

EXPLORING YOUR FLOWS

Remember, subtle energies are not neutral. They carry information and vibrations that contribute to your *web of meaning* — the weave of experience, and expression that you are co-creating with this life in this body.

Thus, dipping into your subtle energies, your flows, your inner dynamics, and learning to work with them becomes a conversation, not just an energy tune-up. You are looking at how you can support your ability to create a more meaningful life.

Shut your eyes and tune in to your body as a whole. Imagine your body is a cup, holding the brew of all that is in your life right now — feeding and nourishing you, demanding your attention, pulling at you, even distorting you with too many stimulants or intoxicants.

Is your cup too full, just right, or not full enough? Feel into it. Is the brew the right one, or does it need to be replaced with an elixir that can support you and sustain you?

If the cup is too full, pick it up and pour off the excess into the Universal Recycling Bin or an off-site storage container. Or give it back to the earth if it would nourish the soil.

If the cup is too empty but has the correct brew, hold out your cup and ask the Universal Supply Team to top you up to the correct level.

And if your cup has the wrong brew, hold it in one hand, and with your other, reach out and request from the Universal Supply Team something more appropriate to replace it with. Once you have received the replacement, empty your cup of the old brew, take at least three deep breaths to feel into the emptiness, then refill your cup with the new brew.

Tune in: What do you feel now, in body, mind, and spirit? When you think about your life, what, if anything, has shifted?

∽ • ∾

Energies don't just move for the sake of moving. They are communicating, exchanging, bringing resources to where they are needed. Therefore, you enhance your support of their movement when you can understand where they live, how they move when healthy, what it feels like when they aren't moving in their best rhythms, and how to influence them.

You can support your energies by interacting with the specific stream that is most relevant to your issue. For example, if you feel your vital energy isn't getting to where you need it, you can go into the distribution stream (page 228) to work specifically on that issue. Or you can address your overall flow, supporting your energies to move in larger, more universal ways. When you notice yourself feeling clogged, for example, or just not at your best, try giving yourself a "Touch Bath" and/or a "Qi Bath" for both overall and localized renewal.

Exercise: Touch Bath, Qi Bath

A "Touch Bath" opens up space and activates your subtle energies to flow more easily. A "Qi Bath" brings in fresh and nourishing energies to refresh your body's subtle flows.

Touch Bath

Tune in to your body as you do this, to notice where you feel congestion or clogged energies or where the energy is low and needs renewal.

Rub your hands together to generate some heat in your fingers. Then, place your hands side by side (or fingertips to fingertips) on your body and, with light to medium pressure, spread them apart at whatever pace feels most comfortable to you. This opens space for energies to flow better in the area under the skin you are spreading. Notice your sensations before and after.

Repeat this motion on your head, face, neck, torso, and legs to open up space everywhere on your body that you can reach.

To open up space on your arms, bunch the thumb and fingertips of one hand together, place them on the opposite arm, and spread them apart on your skin. Repeat in various locations. Or cross your arms and stroke the opposite sides downward from the shoulders, with hands spread open so your fingers can cover as much skin as possible.

Qi Bath

Renew your flow by pulling in vital energies, or qi, from different sources. Reach down to the earth, scoop up *vital earth energy*, and slather it over your skin, like skin cream. Or if you feel your skin can't take it in, repeat the "Touch Bath," but with your hands coated with fresh earth qi. Send it down into your fascia, which will act as a communications array to spread the message of earth energy throughout your body.

Then reach up to the sky to gather in *cosmic energies* emanating from the sun, moon, and stars. Bring those into your "Qi Bath," using your hands to spread and distribute them, via your skin and fascia, anywhere your body is able to receive them.

Pull *love qi* from your heart to spread throughout your whole body, then figure-eight between you and something you love in the world to bring qi from *the beauty of the world* into you. Next, bring in qi from *the waters of life* that hydrate the planet, then dip into *soul juice from your Wiser Self.* Finally, reach for love energy from *the heart of the Divine.* Spread each of these into your body.

Stand still for several moments, breathing deeply, inviting these energies to circulate and spread throughout your body, mind, and spirit.

◌ • ◌

Most spiritual traditions offer maps of some sort to the subtle energies we are made of, because inner explorations generally make these byways more evident to the mind. Whichever of these traditions you wish to explore, I invite you to go beyond learning them with your mind. Take the outside-in explanations of how you are constructed — with meridians or nadis or *doshas* or other structures — and enter them, as I am showing you to enter the streams, so that you can come to know them from the inside out.

Rather than focusing on details from those specific systems, I'd like to guide you in a short exploration of a few more patterns you can discover within your subtle energy movement. And then I'll add more patterns in the coming chapters. We've already addressed figure eights, Celtic weaves, and metabolizing eights in earlier chapters. Now play around also with your circulation of light, your fountain, and your up-down, yin-yang.

◌ Play with It! ◌

The Circulation of Light

Place one hand on your heart chakra and the other on your solar plexus. Breathe in and out, finding a good, slow rhythm that is comfortable for you.

Then sink your attention down into your sacred baton of the self, your energetic spine. You'll find there the *circulation of light*, or micro-cosmic orbit, an energy flow that travels round and round your central core in both directions, along the conception stream and the comprehension flow. Feel into it. With your hand, gently stroke up your midline on the front of your body from your pubic bone to your bottom lip. Then reach around to your back and trace your comprehension flow from the base of your spine up your back as far as you can reach. Next, reach over your shoulder to grab the energy and gently pull it up over the top of your head and down your face, ending at your top lip. This activates both streams to feed the circulation of light around your core.

Then let your hand move in a circular motion, either up the front and down the back or down the front and up the back, feeling into which way your circulation of light is moving in this moment. Try to hook your hand's energy into the circulation of light and let it be pulled like a water skier along in the flow.

You may have to do this physical circling to one side of your body, particularly if you can't reach the back side of the circulation of light. I do this by placing one hand on my heart chakra and using the other hand to trace the circulation of light to the side of my body.

If you can't feel which way the flow is traveling now (it can travel in either or both directions at once), gently use your hand movements to support the flow in one direction, then the other.

The Fountain

Vital qi, a.k.a. earth juice, travels up from the earth through your legs via your Kidney-1 points, located on the soles of each foot, in the slight de-pression created when your foot is pointed downward. This earth qi con-tinues upward via your root chakra; through your energetic spine and body's core, revitalizing all your organs and tissues; then up through your neck and out the top of your head, several feet in the air. (You are happier and more inspired when it is robust, generally feel dull and uninspired when it is not flowing with much oomph.)

Next, like a water fountain, the qi arcs up and out and surrounds you in a large torus shape, a kind of oblong doughnut. The earth juice then rejoins the energy below your feet to return to the earth. When you do the "Porcupine Reset" exercise, one thing it does is reanimate this fountain.

Let your hands travel the pathway of this fountain, tuning in to it and also helping to scoop energies from deep in the earth. Pull them up into your core, then up through your gut, solar plexus, heart, and throat, bathing and revitalizing each of these areas.

Notice where the fountain travels easily and where there is congestion you could clear to help it travel. Support the flow to spring forth from your head, up toward the heavens, then let your hands travel with the flow down to the earth. If you can reach, connect your palms with the earth and listen with your hands as the qi returns to its source under your feet.

If your fountain is not feeling very robust, you can boost it by pulling in energy from your heart, the heart of the Divine, the cosmos, the heart of mother earth, and other sources mentioned on pages 215–16. Trace the pathway of your fountain, infusing it with this booster qi.

The Up-Down, Yin-Yang

As you have learned from tracing the meridian streams, yin energies in general flow (a) from the earth up the body and (b) from the torso out the inside of your arms to your fingertips. Yang flows travel (c) from your fingertips along the backs of your arms to your shoulders and face and also (d) from the top part of your face, over the back of your head, down the back of your body, and off your toes to ground into the earth. The only exception to this is the embodiment flow (stomach meridian, yang), which circles your face like a mask and travels down the front of your body off the second toe to ground you.

Trace this larger yin-yang pattern with open hands. Start with scooping up cosmic energy from the earth, then trace it up the front of your body along your legs and up the front of your torso, from the shoulders out the insides of your arms and hands, and off your finger pads into the web of connections with the larger world.

Then, tracing one arm at a time, pull in energy from the web of connections (or the heavens) into your fingertips, running it along the back of your hand and arm to your shoulder and onto the side of your face.

Finally, trace this flow from your upper face, up over your head, down your back, and off your toes. Return the energy to ground in the earth.

As you trace, feel into whether the energies are freely flowing or sluggish. A body sweep of this sort helps to support the overall circulation of your energies.

☞ • ☜

LIFE FLOW

If you asked her, Carrie would tell you she loved her work. She had recently been promoted and was given expanded oversight of a team of new employees. She truly believed in what she was doing. So she was shocked when she started having difficulty sleeping at night because of jaw pain. Her dentist diagnosed it as TMJ (temporomandibular joint) pain and told her it was caused by stress. Carrie knew she was working harder, but that explanation didn't sound right. She was exhilarated by her new role, so she wasn't sure where the stress was coming from.

She came for an energy assessment to see what she could do to address the TMJ. When she was lying down in a neutral mode, all of her energy systems moved comfortably, and energy tests showed her flow was strong. And when she got up and walked around, her flow also tested strong. But when she walked across the room and I unexpectedly and repeatedly asked her to stop on her way, her body showed us that the stop-start was causing her embodiment stream — the stream that usually governs the TMJ — to fluctuate wildly and the muscles in her jaw to tighten.

Carrie immediately understood what her body was showing us. She admitted that the only part of her new role she didn't like was that the new employees were constantly interrupting her to ask questions, so she had trouble finding any rhythm in her other work.

Once she saw the problem, she could devise solutions, using what I call *lifestyle medicine.* She reworked her schedule to set up predictable office hours. She grouped the new employees in small teams with more experienced folks and encouraged them to problem solve and share information before asking her. She set up daily check-ins for people to ask and answer questions in a contained forum. And she made a Do Not Disturb sign for her door, for moments when she needed to concentrate.

I also taught her to reset her flow using several of the exercises in this chapter. This did the trick; her TMJ and sleep issues disappeared.

When you come to recognize the interplay between your energies and what happens in you physically, you can see that your best medicine can usually be found in how you live, move, use energy, and support or block its flow. And you will recognize that you can address the issue both by working with your streams and other energy flows, using energy medicine, and also by using lifestyle medicine to shift how you live, moment by moment.

WATER AS MEDICINE, WATER AS TEACHER

I remember the first time I heard someone say that water, especially access to clean water, was rapidly becoming the number one challenge confronting our world. It was in the late-1980s in Hong Kong. People at international child development conferences and UN gatherings I was involved in increasingly named water as the highest priority to focus on. At first, I was taken aback by this. In the midst of discussions of violence, poverty, wars, human trafficking, air pollution, and other world-threatening topics, why would access to clean water jump to the head of the list?

But then I realized it is because water is our lifeblood, vital to our existence. We can't last much more than three days without it: it regulates our temperature, our internal communications, the health of our cells. Since we are mostly water (our blood is 90 percent water, our cells are 60 percent, and our bones are 31 percent), it is clearly crucial to our very survival.

And that is true for the larger body of the planet as well: 71 percent of our mother earth is covered in water. The movement and circulation of waters — underground, via waterways and surface bodies, and through the processes of evaporation and precipitation — regulate the very health of the planet.

When we talk about someone being out of their element, we use the phrase "like a fish out of water." But in fact, we might as well say "like a human out of water"!

There is much we can learn from water itself, as an element within us and around us. Consider some qualities of water:

- Water *enlivens* us, and plants, and planet earth.
- Water *conducts* energy, sound, and other vibrations.

- Water *transports* nutrients.
- Water *travels* via conduits (streams) and osmosis.
- Water *gathers and gains mass* in containers.
- Water *saturates and hydrates* whatever it can access.

Water is a wonderful model to help us understand subtle energies. Like water, your energies can freeze (get sluggish), flow, expand like a gas or concentrate like a solid, and behave like "tunneling water" (which in tight spaces creates quantum channels and takes on never-before-seen shapes!). Like water, subtle energy both shapes and is shaped by the other elements; it travels through conduits, such as the meridian streams, or diffuses via saturation in energy fields such as the aura. Like water, subtle energy gains mass when contained and will travel wherever it can get access.

Water conducts energy and facilitates communication in your body, mind, and spirit. That's why taking time to sip water or immersing yourself in a bath can activate healing.

∾ Play with It! ∾

My Councils introduced the concept of water as medicine early in our work together. Fill a small glass with water. Hold the glass in your hands and infuse into it whatever medicine you believe you need.

I usually put in an energetic form of whatever I'm looking for, rather than putting in specific chemical signatures. For example, I infuse the water with an energetic calmer, muscle relaxer, wound healer, blood cleanser, or even an antibiotic or antifungal. Or if I am not certain what is needed, I ask the Universal Supply Team (or the Divine) for the perfect essence to resolve my energetic challenge, and I infuse that into the water.

Occasionally I make my own homemade "homeopathic," bringing a specific chemical signature to the water. Note: if you are taking pharmaceuticals your body is dependent on, work with a licensed health care practitioner to figure out how to experiment with the homemade version responsibly.

You can infuse the water with emotional or spiritual medicine as well: gratitude, peace, acceptance, kindness.

Then slowly sip the water, feeling it carry the message you have infused into it to every cell in your body, activating the communication in the water residing in your cells, your bones, your blood.

I have used this technique for nearly fifty years, and it has saved me time and again from having to go the chemical route to invite my body's functions to shift and heal.

◌ • ◌

Gina woke up tired every morning and felt like she was gasping for energy, the way you gasp for breath. She could barely drag herself out of bed and into her day. She just couldn't get plugged into whatever juice she was supposed to have to run her body.

And that caused her to feel anxiety. So within about an hour, she'd find herself alternating between being exhausted and tapped out to feeling frantic, jangly, and overjuiced, like she was being electrocuted.

She couldn't figure out if she needed more energy or less. And she couldn't figure out what would help. All day long she kept swinging from crashed out to overjazzed.

Her naturopath told her she was suffering from adrenal fatigue and gave her several supplements to boost her adrenals. Her MD tested her for thyroid issues, and her blood work came back showing her thyroid was mildly off-kilter. They decided to check it again in six months.

But meanwhile, Gina was barely functioning. She felt as though the problem was spiraling and getting worse.

In fact, both practitioners were right...and not quite right. Gina's glands were affected because her energy relays were not working properly. In carrying out the work of your body, your energies need to collaborate and flow from one to another. The energy relays act a bit like the flippers in an old-fashioned pinball machine — opening, closing, working together to send your energies traveling through your system to fuel what needs to be juiced. And if the relay is off-kilter, then that can cause your adrenals, your thyroid, your hypothalamus, the pineal and pituitary glands in your head, your blood sugar metabolism, your burners, and other parts of the relay system to over- and underperform.

Often when we are diagnosed with glandular issues we can heal these without needing to medicate if we work with the energetics and the relays involved.

In order to heal, Gina needed to partner with her water element streams — the element that supports and maintains flow in the body — and with her gatekeeper, which maintains or interferes with the relays that allocate resources as needed.

She used the "Electrics Eye Hold" to calm her nervous system, which is governed by water element.

Exercise: Electrics Eye Hold

The electrical activities of the brain can keep overstimulating the energetic spine (and keep thoughts spinning their wheels in our head). This eye hook-up hold can help.

Close your eyes and place your index finger, without pressing, on your upper eyelid toward the edge of the eye. Place your middle finger on your eye socket, the bony surround on the outside of your eye (see figure 11.1). If possible, do this two-finger hold on both eyes at once. As with most hook-ups, hold it until you feel calming, a release, or another signal to stop.

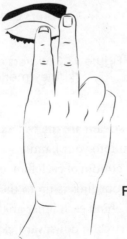

Figure 11.1. Electrics Eye Hold

◌ • ◌

To partner with her gatekeeper, Gina worked with her four chambers (pages 123–26), reset her yin relay using "Gatekeeper Syncing" (pages 116–17), and reset her yang relay using the "Energy Relay Reset" (pages 114–16).

And then she visited both of her water element streams to reinstate the natural rhythms of her flow.

Tracing the Waters of Life Stream (Kidney Meridian)

High Tide: 5 p.m. to 7 p.m.
Element: Water
Direction: Yin
Trace this stream on both the left and right sides of your body.

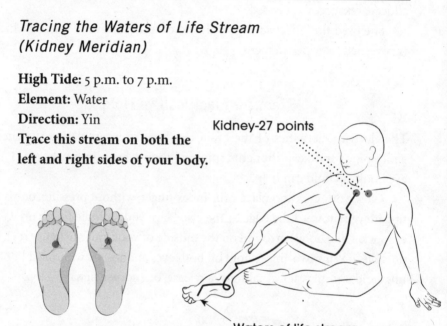

Figure 11.2. Kidney-1 points

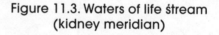

Figure 11.3. Waters of life stream (kidney meridian)

The cosmic sources for this stream are the waters under the surface of the earth. Scoop them into your hands.

Place your fingers on the bottom of each foot, in the K-1 points (see figure 11.2). Now, draw your fingers up to the inner edges of each foot, and trace a circle behind each inner ankle bone, tracing upward near the bone, and circling downward closer to the heel (see figure 11.3). You're making a clockwise circle from front to back on the right foot and a counterclockwise circle on the left foot.

Then trace straight up the inside of the leg. Continue up the front of the body to the two K-27 points beneath the collarbone at the top of the sternum, about one inch on either side of the midline. Vigorously massage or thump these points.

Guided Visit: Waters of Life Stream

The cosmic sources for this stream are the waters that renew and resuscitate the earth — moving underground, traveling over her surface, and existing within our environment.

The waters of life stream is the flow that brings in vital qi, or life force energy — the energy that feeds all the other streams. And its emotion is hope. Think of the phrase "Hope springs eternal." Its cosmic source is the waters of the earth, the springs, the damp, the rivers and lakes and oceans, the moisture patterns in weather, all moving in constant cycles of renewal.

This stream feeds your inner sense of knowing, your inner confidence and sense of self, and is also a wellspring of creativity. It is a place to come to just float and dream, to experience death and rebirth, or to close others out of the room so you can hear your own truth. It is a place to come to find balance — between yin and yang, between being and doing. To find renewal.

It is here that your being pulls in the vital energy to build bones, to create hormones, to fuel and nourish the operations of your Earth Elemental Self, to support your ability to hear, both literally and figuratively.

Trace the stream with your hands, using the instructions above.

Get comfortable where you are lying or sitting down and shut your eyes. Breathe in and out, in and out, feeling the rise and fall, the ancient rhythm of receiving and releasing, the yin and yang built into your instrument. Place one hand just below your collarbone, covering the two end points of this stream. Tap a slow drumbeat rhythm on these points, echoing what you imagine is the drumbeat of the earth.

Choose a point along this stream, on either side of your body, where you can shrink yourself down to enter the stream or sink your attention down into the flow. Use all your senses to tune in to this place. What do you notice about it? What do you hear, feel, see, smell, taste, sense, or know about it?

What waters do you find here? Are they moving or still? Vibrant or placid? Are they contained, perhaps by the banks of the stream or other retainers, or are they flowing unchecked? How deep are these waters?

What is your instinct about interacting with this stream? Do you want to dip into the water, sit beside it, walk along its pathway, find a protected place from which to experience it? Listen to your instincts and explore as is comfortable for you.

If the place is polluted or the water needs filtering or dredging to remove obstructions or impurities, call upon the Universal Supply Team to help you get it cleared. And if you aren't sure what it requires, ask the stream what it needs from you and then turn that guidance over to the Universal Supply Team to set in motion.

If you are comfortable, just sit or lie back somewhere in this space and let yourself enter into reverie, floating in the unknown for a time. Let your mind just wander, noticing what arises but not trying to control or direct it. Breathe in and out and just notice what your mind does as you release it to wander...and breathe...and feel yourself supported where you are sitting or lying or floating.

Remember this place, because you can come back here for rest and renewal as you need it.

Invite all your past and future selves to join you here beside or within the waters of life stream. Arrange these selves in a figure eight around you, with your past selves on one half of the eight, your future selves on the other, and you in this life at the crossover point. Invite these selves to hold hands. Then send a beloved color, a truest wish, or a note that seems to represent your spirit around the eight in a big wave of affirmation. Feel it traveling around the eight. Feel each self squeezing the hand of the being next to them in turn, until you sense the impulse traveling evenly and easily through the entire figure eight. This will help the life force energy to flow throughout your whole being and will support your many selves to find common cause and shared vision.

Now, place one hand on your heart and the other hand on your two K-27 points below your collarbone. Breathe in and out and choose a place to exit the stream, bringing your awareness fully into your body as it is sitting or lying down in your room. Invite the vital qi you experienced in the waters of life stream to seep wherever it is needed in your body and mind. Open your eyes.

Take a moment to jot down what you experienced here.

∽ • ∽

Tracing Distribution Stream (Bladder Meridian)

High Tide: 3 p.m. to 5 p.m.
Element: Water
Direction: Yang
Trace this stream on both the left and right sides of your body.

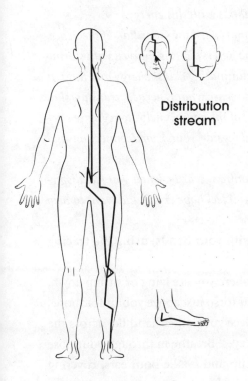

Distribution
stream

Reach out to gather in beauty from the world and fill your hands with awe to activate the cosmic flow.

This stream has two branches.

Branch one: Placing both hands between your eyebrows, trace up over the crown of your head and down the back of your head and neck (see figure 11.4).

Removing your hands from your neck, reach them back and as high up your upper back as you can, stretching along the sides of your spine. Send your intention up to the top of the spine to pull the energy down.

Now, trace down both sides of your spine to below your waist, jog in and up toward the waist again, and then trace down

Figure 11.4. Distribution stream (bladder meridian)

and circle them around your gluteus maximus, following the contours of your buttocks.

Branch two: Leaving that branch, place your hands on your shoulders. Then reach around back again, as high as you can, to catch the meridian energy and pull it straight down your back and the backs of your legs to your knees. Jog in at the knees, then trace further along the backs of your legs down to the floor and off your little toes.

Guided Visit: Distribution Stream

The cosmic source of this distribution stream filters into the body through your aura to enrich your senses. Reach out to gather in the beauty of sight and sound and sensation and fill your hands with this energy.

The distribution flow is also sometimes called the Guardian of the Peace, the Great Mediator, or the Minister of the Reservoir. It is charged with storing and distributing vital qi and fluid and eliminating excess energy and fluid. It communicates via your nervous system to sense what is needed, translate that into action, and integrate the operations of the body. It helps to regulate electrical communications in your body, alongside your heart/connection and comprehension streams.

This stream is a place to come to confront fear or when you feel dispirited, but it is also a place to visit when you feel hope rising and want to help yourself release the old and birth the new.

Trace your distribution stream with your hands, using the tracing instructions above.

Close your eyes, get comfortable where you are lying or sitting down, and place one hand on the front of your torso just above your pubic bone, over your bladder. If you can reach, place your other hand flat across the back of your head, at the level of your eyes. Breathe in through your nose and out through your mouth. Now cup and cradle both ears, covering them with your palms, and hold for three deep breaths.

Using your index and middle fingers, do an "Electrics Eye Hold"

(page 223) for at least three deep breaths, lightly touching your closed eyelid with one finger and the bony surround of your eye with the other.

Now, choosing an entry point somewhere along the distribution
stream we traced, shrink yourself down or sink your attention down into
the flow. Use all your senses to explore where you have landed: What
do you hear, see, smell, taste, or feel in this place? Pay attention to what
thoughts arise in your mind and how comfortable it is for you here.

Because it is such a long stream and it deals with distribution, you
may want to take soundings at several places to get a sense of where the
flow is moving or impeded and how healthy it is. Visit the stream as it
travels over your head, at the double branches along your spine, in your
legs and feet.

Now, find a place along your spine where you can assess more specifically the energy in this flow.

Invite the Guardian of the Peace, the keeper of this stream, to come
sit with you here. What is needed to make this a place of hope and affirmation? Ask them what they particularly want you to know, right now, in
order for you to find greater balance in your yin and yang, your receiving
and releasing.

Thank them for any insights they give you and call upon the Universal
Supply Team to do any repairs or adjustments needed in this distribution
stream.

Now, if you are not already in the area of your spine, bring your attention to that portion of the stream. We are going to walk through clearing
and anchoring your sacred baton of the self as you sit or lie here in deeper
communion with your distribution stream.

Bend the fingers of each hand as though preparing to play the piano.
Bring your hands down to the base of your torso in front, where your
bladder organ sits. Behind it is the base of your spine. Place one bent hand
on each side of your midline about two to three inches apart, the same
distance they would be on your back if they were placed between the bony
processes of your spine.

Open up your fingertips to stream out laser beams of colored light.
Tune in to the portion of the spine your hands are covering and open to
whatever you can perceive about the nerves in that area. Are they sluggish

or active? Signaling smoothly or erratically? Is there anything clogging the area?

Use the colored lights streaming from your fingertips to clear out any blockages and to reset the energies in that area of your spine. If you wish to then send the lights through to anchor somewhere, let them seek anchorage and stay open to picking up a confirmation signal, maybe a voice that says, "We have you" or a sense of clicking into place, of landing.

Then move your bent fingers up your midline, covering the next bit of energetic spine, around the level of your belly button. Again, tune in to that area, opening your attention to the nerves that run through there. Are they working smoothly or struggling? Is there anything clogging their function?

Remember, you can always ask the Universal Supply Team to help repair nerves and even bone. But also, turn on your colored laser lights, stream them from your fingers, and use them to reset the connections and retune the frequencies of the energies in that area of your spine. If you wish, send the lights further to anchor and notice if you get a sense of arrival, a confirmation.

Again, move your hands, fingers bent, upward to cover the next portion of your energetic spine, around your solar plexus. Tune in and investigate the energies you find there. Your goal in this work is to clear, reset, and tune the distribution system of nerves and vital life force energy emanating from your spine. Send the laser lights in to clear and reconnect and then onward to anchor and ground you.

Move your hands upward again, with fingers bent, landing around your heart area. Tune in to the energies in the stream you find here and send your laser lights in to untangle and clean up the distribution of qi through this crucial, very electric area. Use your laser lights to open up space in your back and seek anchorage and grounding.

Again move upward, to your upper chest, and place your bent fingers on either side of the midline. Tune in to the distribution stream here — what do you notice? Activate your colored laser lights to open up space, remove any excess, and energize the area. And then allow the beams to travel through and seek anchorage and grounding. Listen for the signal of connection.

And, finally, bring your bent fingers to your throat, straddling the midline, and tune in to the energies in this area of the stream. Allow your colored laser lights to activate and gently clear out, disentangle, open up, and support the energies traveling through this area. Send the laser lights out through the back of your neck to seek anchorage and grounding. Listen for the signal that they have been received.

Now, bring your hands up to your eyes and once again do a two-finger "Electrics Eye Hold," with one finger on your closed eyelid and the other on the bony surround. You can do this for one eye or both. And breathe.

Then, lightly cup both ears with your hands, sending warmth and love and the vital energy of this stream in to clear and clean out your entire hearing apparatus. And breathe.

And then place one palm on the back of your head behind your eyes and the other at the base of your torso over the bladder, above your pubic bone. Hold them there for three deep breaths, in through your nose and out through your mouth.

And when you feel ready, exit the stream at any point along its pathway. Open your eyes and bring your attention back to the room.

Take a moment to jot down anything you noticed.

∞ • ∞

I must admit that I just love watching a time-lapse rendition of a plant unfolding from a seed, a puppy growing into doghood, a baby traveling from birth to death, a weather event unfolding: spirit flowing from form to form. Change happens, and it can illuminate our minds and hearts — renew us — to experience positive evolution and even much-needed deaths and rebirths over time.

But when change messes with your rhythms, pacing, ability to move or find space to move, it will often trigger your gatekeeper, unground you, wipe out your glue, and interfere with your capacity to flow as you are designed to flow. When change triggers your gatekeeper, it drains your power to adapt physically or emotionally or warps your understandings of the world. This will impact your map of meaning, the canvas of self you are creating in this life as a soul having a human experience.

As change in the world as we know it keeps accelerating, learning how to work with flow is increasingly valuable. In chapter 12, "Your Web of Meaning," we'll look at how to use the streams and energy tools to work with larger flow to support your creation of meaning in this life.

⚭ Chapter Twelve ⚭

Your Web of Meaning

Why is one person enlivened by a 1964 GI Joe doll and another by discovering a new form of fungus? Why do I love plastic cups (true confession) while my friend will drink only from glass? It is because, as souls having an experience in this shared earth reality, we are each weaving a personalized web of meaning. What is meaningful to me might mean bupkis to you.

Your web of meaning is more than just a catalog of personal preferences. Meaning supports flow: it motivates you to act and choose; it animates your weave of energies. Your web of meaning feeds you and nourishes your body, your mind, and your spirit in quite individualized ways.

When given a choice, I choose to pursue a particular line of work, because doing that work enlivens me, gives my life validity. And I organize my time, belongings, and actions in certain ways, because doing so gives significance to my effort and feeds my web of meaning.

I think of my web of meaning as an energetic backup battery, a place where my gatekeeper stores energy generated from anything that touches my soul, moves me, animates me, feeds me.

I'm not talking about substances that stimulate you, like coffee, but rather about experiences that strike the gong of your nature, gratify, and nourish you in direct, visceral ways.

In your energy systems, you have a feature my Councils call your *safety net* (Donna Eden calls it your *minor grid*), where your web of meaning gets stored. In a time when nothing is particularly nourishing me, I can recall that beautiful sunset that left me trembling with awe, can draw on the faith that you still love me even though you've been too busy to see me for the past week, can know I deserve to receive love and to be alive, even if it isn't apparent in this moment — *because I have resources stored in my safety net to use as backup.*

Care and feeding of your web of meaning and of your safety net are investments in inner resilience.

WHEN YOUR WEB OF MEANING GETS DAMAGED

Kingston was a successful real estate broker and worked long hours to serve his clients, who raved about how good he was at his job. And that meant something to him. But because he pretty much worked most of his waking hours, he had trouble finding a partner who would stay with him longer than a year or two. And although he worked out regularly at a gym to get buff, he was not really at ease in his body.

When he injured his shoulder, he had to take a break from his workout routine and to cut back on driving, which hobbled his work. As a result, he experienced a sudden emotional and energetic crash. He described it as not knowing what to do with himself. As if some vital cord was cut that had previously kept him in the flow of his life.

In short order, he found himself assailed by doubts, unhappy with work that had pleased him a month earlier, and in general unsure why he should get up in the morning and keep going. A friend urged him to see a psychotherapist, but he decided to check out energy medicine instead, because he had seen a video online that mentioned it could help with vitality, pain, and wound healing.

As he suspected, Kingston's experience involved his emotions, but the feelings he was having emanated from energetic causes. When he injured his shoulder, he also bruised his web of meaning, tore the part of it that relates to being anchored and connected. So he had a *grounding* issue. The injury also interrupted his sense of purpose, which left him feeling unglued and lacking *coherence.* And, of course, that sense of having his life derailed caused a major interruption to the energetic *flow* within his web of meaning.

Emotions are wonderful indicators of what is happening with your energies. I am not the first person to notice that the word *e-motion* could be a contraction for "energy in motion." But often the feelings that arise in the midst of a change are *symptoms* of disrupted energetic dynamics rather than the *causes* of the disruption we are feeling. So it is worth your while to do what you can to address the energy dynamics underlying your feelings, whether or not you also seek out counseling.

When Kingston heard about his web of meaning, his first reaction was, "Bingo!" He said, "I know this injury is here to teach me something. I should not feel this derailed by having to change my routine." He could see that he needed to work on supporting and extending his web of meaning. This meant seeking out experiences that would touch him and strike the gong of his nature.

To repair his damaged safety net, he learned the following technique.

Protocol: Epicenter Repair

An epicenter is a bruise on your web of meaning that causes an energy vortex to form, which then either pulls you repeatedly to similar experiences or calls similar experiences to you. The purpose of this is to give you opportunities to learn and grow. But sometimes the vortex just wounds you further or creates pain and illness in the energies or parts of the body that relate to where the vortex has formed.

Think about a stream with a sizable boulder in it. Where the boulder breaks the surface, the waters swirl around it, forming a vortex. Your energies do the same thing around a tear in your safety net.

To locate an epicenter, use a four-finger notch (thumb plus index, middle, and fourth fingers bunched together) to feel into your safety net in places where you suspect your net has been disrupted. I see your safety net as covering not only your physical body, but also your aura. However, it is generally most potent in the area covered by your body weave (pages 201–3). When I use my four-finger notch, I always think of those electrical probes electricians use to find active circuits.

If you know how to energy test yourself or if you are working with a practitioner who uses energy tests, touch the suspect area with your four-finger notch while testing the energy. A weak test shows there is an epicenter in that area. (See appendix A for instructions on how to energy test.)

You can also do the "Body Weave" and use your four-finger notch to probe for places where the weave is disrupted and needs epicenter repair.

If you find one epicenter on your safety net, know there are often other places that also need to be repaired. This is because a pull or damage to the tension of the weave often torques and affects the overall net.

Pay attention to moments when it seems like history is repeating itself in habitual thoughts, actions, events, or symptoms. These are likely to indicate you have a bruise on your web of meaning and need to do some epicenter healing!

To repair an epicenter, draw the five-element star and circle on the area where you found the epicenter, either directly on the skin or just above it (see figure 12.1). Figure-eight at least three times each between water and fire, fire and metal, metal and wood, wood and earth, earth and water. Then trace a clockwise circle (as if figure 12.1 were printed on that

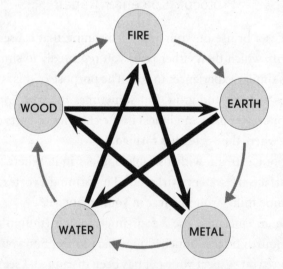

Figure 12.1. Tracing the five-pointed star and circle

area of your body). Do this slowly and lovingly, while focusing on the issue that seems related to the bruise, if you know it.

This exercise reinstates the balance of elements and flow in the area. Often it will release the energy vortex and associated emotions as well.

∽ • ∾

To strengthen and support his safety net, Kingston used the "Body Weave" exercise several times a day, followed by a simple exercise I call the "Harmonizing Hook-Up" (introduced in my book *The Language Your Body Speaks*). It is worth repeating here, because it supports flow from the inside out.

Exercise: Harmonizing Hook-Up

This exercise strengthens your safety net and helps to integrate your various energy flows. It is good for resetting your perspective to a more balanced state.

Place one palm flat on the front of your left shoulder, where your arm connects to your torso, and the other palm flat on the front of your left pelvis/hip. Imagine yourself being held in the arms of the Divine or rocked in a rainbow hammock. (You can rock in a literal rainbow hammock if you have one.) Open yourself to the heavens and earth. Hold these hand positions in silence for about three minutes, allowing your energies to harmonize.

This is particularly rich to have someone do for you. Your partner would open their feet and head to the earth and sky, place their hands on your left shoulder and left pelvis/hip area, and hold in silence for at least three minutes while you hold hands with the Divine.

∽ • ∾

CARE AND FEEDING OF YOUR WEB OF MEANING

As I have said before, energy medicine is enhanced when paired with life-style medicine. If, like Kingston, your web of meaning is being nourished only in limited realms (work and exercise, for him), then exploring and expanding your range of what strikes the gong of your nature becomes your new best medicine.

When you take the risk to love — and love widely — objects, moments, words, thoughts, artworks, people, and creatures in their quirky, infinite variety, you strengthen your safety net, your resilience, and your store of inner resources.

And your secret superpower in this endeavor is *curiosity*. If that has disappeared from your lexicon, whip up some water medicine infused with curiosity and sip it while inviting your body to show you in your mind's screening room at least one new thing you'd like to explore.

THE SHARED WEB OF MEANING

We don't live in a vacuum. Although we each have an individual and unique web of meaning, we also collectively assign shared significance to experiences and choices. These are often culture specific. In one culture, it is considered meaningful to serve the collective in an unobtrusive way; in another culture, value comes from distinguishing yourself from the crowd. In one culture, formal education might bring enrichment and deepen your experience; in another, it can be considered a betrayal of traditional values or group membership.

When the shared web of meaning also feeds you personally, that can be a plus. Consider the individuals who feel glory when their favorite sports team wins the championship. Consider the television show that awakens your compassion and sense of collective membership with a story about people who might not even exist in real life.

But it becomes problematic when the shared web of meaning demands your time, energy, and allegiance or torques your ability to appreciate your own experience. Like the person so desperate to marry because it is the norm, they can't appreciate the ways that flying solo feeds them. Like the person who can't appreciate her love of swimming, because she's convinced it is valuable only if she excels. Like Kingston, who bought into the notion that working so hard to be successful is good — in a field that defines success by volume of sales rather than personal fulfillment. He paid for it with malnourishment in his safety net.

WORKING WITH YOUR STREAMS IS AN ART FORM

Streams emanate from cosmic sources. In a way, you could say they are cosmic flows, cosmic nourishment. They are also the specific energetic vibrations that your body uses to create your physical instrument and mind.

My Old Chinese Gentleman used to insist that I enter the streams, over and over again, to understand and work with what was going on energetically inside my clients. He also had dozens of ways to name the various flavors of stream energy. As Chinese medicine got adopted and translated in the West, the meridian names lost their poetry; they were flattened and standardized, mostly to the name of the organ they serve — spleen, gallbladder, liver. Contrast the name "spleen" with "Minister of the Granary." By using organ names we have lost much of the understanding of the energies in each stream.

That's one reason I chose to rename/reframe the meridians and call them streams, giving them names that start to capture a bit of their essence. But I encourage you to build on these and expand your nicknames for each flow.

The stream names I've provided throughout this book — energizer, yin protector, heart/connection, choice/discernment, conception, comprehension, nourishment, embodiment, purpose, enactor/enforcer, give and receive, distiller/refiner, waters of life, and distribution — make up a starter kit to support you in getting to know these energies as the paints on your palette, the threads in your weave, the notes on your musical scale. The goal is to become an artist of using these core energies in healing the self you have created and creating the self you want to bring forth.

I see the streams as a place to unpack and develop meaning, a place to influence the distribution of resources, a place to work from the inside out on my health and life (and to support my clients in their evolution).

In allopathic medicine, we consider it quite normal to analyze blood in order to diagnose illness or body function. And we then think it's reasonable to use pharmaceuticals to influence the blood and the body's chemical communications.

So why would many people doubt that you can both recognize and address illness by working with your streams? The streams are like your energetic blood, and when you visit them regularly, you will start to feel it is normal to work with them not only to gain insights into your energetic makeup but also to address illness and support your overall construction of self, the flow of your consciousness into form.

How Do You Know Which Stream to Enter When?

1. Let your hand show you. Scan your body with your hand and see where you are drawn to give support. Then enter the stream that either is nearest to that area or relates to the organ your hand is nearest.

2. Intuit or energy test which of the elements needs support now and visit the associated streams:

   - **Water** = distribution (yang); waters of life (yin)
   - **Wood** = enactor/enforcer (yang); purpose (yin)
   - **Fire** = choice/discernment, energizer (yang); heart/connection, yin protector (yin)
   - **Earth** = embodiment (yang); nourishment (yin)
   - **Metal** = distiller/refiner (yang); give and receive (yin)
   - **Air** = conception and comprehension

   To enhance clear intuition, use an "ambassador" from each element: a glass of water, a growing plant for wood, flame, a stone for earth, a metal object, and a fan or your own breath for air. Hold each ambassador in turn near your solar plexus or center and tune in to see whether your body needs the support of that element now.

   If you know how to energy test, a simple way to do this is to hold the ambassador to your solar plexus and say, "Show me a weak test if this element needs support," then energy test.

Then visit at least one of the streams related to the weak element. In general, it makes some sense to go first to the yin stream of that element, because supporting the yin often calms the yang. But use your instincts about where to go first or visit both the yin and yang streams.

3.   Tune in to see what energy issues are coming up for you. Talk to friends about your discomforts and challenges and listen to the language you are using. Once you recognize which energy dynamics are at the forefront, you can enter the streams that relate to those issues:

- **Gatekeeping:** issues of safety, identity, energy distribution/allocation, or habits. Work with the fire streams.
- **Grounding:** issues of release, rooting/nourishment, centering, or anchoring. Work with the earth streams and the conception and comprehension streams.
- **Coherence:** issues with purpose / guiding vision, connectors/glue, structure/container that unifies, or integration / getting in sync. Work with the wood streams and metal streams.
- **Flow:** Issues with sourcing qi from cosmic sources, distribution and delivery of qi, circulation, or influencing flow. Work with the water streams.

4.   See appendix B, "Which Stream Do I Visit When?," for reminders of the cosmic sources and possible reasons for entering each stream.

A Visitor's Guide to the Streams: How Can You Influence Them?

1.   **Visit them.** Take a quick dip in to see what you perceive, to listen and learn.
2.   **Trace the flow with your hand.** Backward tracing clears the energy; forward tracing strengthens and supports it. A good pattern is to trace backward one or two times, then forward three or more times.

3. **Use gauges.** Go into your mental control room and find a dial or gauge labeled with the name of this stream. Adjust the flow to normal or whatever setting you desire.

4. **Use water as medicine.** Hold a glass of water and energetically infuse it with something the stream needs — a purifier, a calmer, a collector, an unblocker, or some positive quality, such as grace. Infuse that water with the quality, then sip it slowly while focused on the energy stream you want to influence, or else dip into the infused water with your fingers and draw along the path of your stream. (This also works with other substances, like homeopathics or Bach flower remedies.)

5. **Make up a gesture or movement** that activates, balances, shifts, calms, or integrates the energies of a stream. Tap, massage, figure-eight, or pulse along the pathway. Or use a whole-body exercise while focusing on the flow, like tossing a beanbag back and forth from one hand to another or doing the "Porcupine Reset."

6. **Use energy dialogue to influence flow.** Speak to the stream using all your senses. Send music through the stream; shine a colored light along the pathway; or wrap it in colored cloth. Use tapping plus rhythm; bathe it in sunshine or moonshine; trace sacred shapes along it, such as hearts or the five-element star and circle (page 236).

7. **Entrain with a healthier flow.** Align yourself with a stronger or higher vibration energy or with another person whose flow is working well. This is a form of energy overlay.

8. **Spin a magnet or crystal over it.** Using a cut glass crystal or magnet on a string helps the polarities to rebalance. You can also flip your hand back and forth, front and back, over the stream.

9. **Unclog.** Grab clogged energy and pull it out of your field. Or use sound to unclog a flow.

10. **Do symbolic clearing.** Visit the stream to clear rocks or other debris with the help of the Universal Supply Team.

11. **Filter the energy.** Use a screen, as in the "Spinal Fluid Screen" exercise (pages 162–63), to remove impurities.

12. **Find energetic antidotes** that shift everything. Use your intuition for what might work or see if something in range pops into your consciousness. For example, if the stream seems too acidic, pour in some energetic alkaline.

13. **Rework the containers.** Water needs a container — so does energy! You can work on the streambeds, putting in dams or earthworks.

14. **Juice the system.** Dip into the cosmic flows to juice your flows.

15. **Strengthen the circulation of all the flows.** To support the circulation, you can trace all the meridians in order. Donna Eden teaches individual meridian tracing in a circuit, enabling you to explore the entire system of streams and their patterns of flow. You can learn this helpful skill from the "Tracing Meridians with Donna Eden" video on YouTube (youtu.be /Vv5dkvMg1z4). Or work with the streams that feed, control, are fed by, or are controlled by the flow you wish to influence, as detailed in table 12.1 below.

ELEMENTS ARE YOUR TEACHERS

You already have a vast store of knowledge about elements and how they influence you.

You know water in its many forms: wet and runny, slushy or steamy, and everything in between. You know its behaviors and qualities. You know that if you are underwater, you can't see very clearly or breathe. You know that if you are on top of water, you can float. You know that if you are immersed in water, you are not as heavy as it is, and you'll move more lightly than in air but also more slowly.

And you know the difference between water and wood (and other plant forms). You know all kinds of things about how plants grow and behave, about the growth factor that characterizes the wood element.

And you do not have any trouble distinguishing wood from fire or the behaviors of each. Nor do you confuse fire and earth or earth and metal. And air does not ever confuse you into thinking it is earth, metal, fire, wood, or even water, though it can feel wet like water if you are in a mist, since that is a mixture of air and water.

So the elements already form a rich energetic vocabulary for you.

And you know that if you water a plant, it grows; if you feed a tree to the fire, it burns brighter; if you shine light on the earth, it becomes capable of sustaining life; if you enclose metal minerals in earth, they become condensed and solid; if you create a pot for water, it is held and supported.

Back in the early days of Chinese medicine, in the era my Old Chinese Gentleman hails from, it was these relationships between elements that formed the basis for understanding the interrelationships between the streams. It was an inside-out way of knowing the energies, rooted in everyday, natural experience.

Water feeds wood but is supported or fed by metal in the form of containers. And water controls fire by damping its ardor. Water is controlled by earth in the form of riverbanks, dams, and mud that slows it down. These were just logical, commonplace understandings of energy.

Table 12.1. The relationships among the elements

Element Relationships				
Element	Feeds	Is Fed By	Controls	Is Controlled By
Water	Wood	Metal	Fire	Earth
Wood	Fire	Water	Earth	Metal
Fire	Earth	Wood	Metal	Water
Earth	Metal	Fire	Water	Wood
Metal	Water	Earth	Wood	Fire

Where does the element of air fit into this thinking? It blows in to influence the yin and yang of each element. Wind whips up or puts out fire; wind blows earth asunder or fertilizes it with gentle movement. Wind moves water or disperses it. Wind supports trees to release excess foliage or blows them over. Wind shears metal or sets it resonating. The air element sits in the central corridor of the conception and comprehension streams or sometimes is best encountered in the give and receive stream, which governs the lungs.

∽ Play with It! ∽

Choose a stream to enter. Base your choice on the energy issue you want to address, which pathway your pain sits closest to, which organ needs support, or what your intuition tells you. Go spend some time there or listen to a Guided Visit (download the corresponding MP3 recording at ellenmeredith.com/visits, password: YBSW). When you feel complete, jot down what you experienced or learned.

Then look at table 12.1 and find the element of your chosen stream in the far-left column. Explore a stream that is related to the element that feeds your stream, that is fed by your stream, that controls your stream, and that is controlled by your stream.

Gather insights and keep track of what these related flows can teach you about your issue and about the energy stream — the energetic strand of your web of meaning — that you are aiming to support.

∽ • ∽

When you can transcend the flattening and distortion of our outside-in culture and really leap into the language of energy with both feet and both hands, you have ways to participate in initiating change and in navigating the changes that happen to you and around you. The streams offer a rich palette of energies to work with as you step up to participate more fully in creating your self. Working with flow gives you ways to engage with your own moving, shifting patterns of energies from the inside out.

Furthermore, you can apply what you know about the elements and streams and energies to events in the world around you. You will begin to recognize when an interaction needed more heart energy or less distiller energy. You will see how a larger social event is unbalanced in its fire or wood element.

In the following two chapters, I explore the larger dynamics of change: exchange between self and world (also known as your *web of connections*) and radiance, the soul juice that animates all that we are and do.

∽ Chapter Thirteen ∾

The Web of Connections

When we talk about teaching kids about the birds and the bees, we usually mean sex. But there's another lesson here that may be more important than procreation. It's about how we are all inter-connected, like the birds and the bees. All life-forms, all of consciousness is inter-connected in what my Councils call "the web of connections." They brought this up at the very start of my training: "Each of you is here in this life to work on two things: your web of meaning and your participation in the web of connections."

Evidence of the web of connections is all around us in nature. We see the birds flying in flocks, not crashing into one another, often cooperating to support individuals within their flight. And we observe bees working in hives, complex forms of communal living. We hear whales communicating underwater and witness the mysteries of long-distance migrations of various species. We know that the fungal world communicates via the mycelium and trees via their roots. Swarm consciousness is all over nature.

And yet somehow we tend to live as though we are blind to our inter-connections with the ecology of life-forms and to our built-in capacity to participate in the web of connections.

The fifth aspect of working with change (after *gatekeeping, grounding, coherence,* and *flow*) is understanding *exchange between self and world.* You are designed to participate in both social and energetic exchanges. If you fall out of the web of connections or your exchanges are blocked, distorted, or carrying energies that don't support you to thrive, you can quickly get sick and lose perspective. Most chronic illnesses, and many of the larger social problems we seem unable to solve, are rooted in skewed or distorted participation in the web of connections.

This phenomenon has been made startlingly clear with the advent of the internet and World Wide Web, both amazingly evocative names if webworking is part of our deepest purpose! All the patterns of successful swarm behavior (the crowd collaborating to help an individual in trouble or appreciate someone's talent) and toxic swarm behavior (bullying and the spread of disinformation and ungrounded "truths") have been made visible to us.

In a way, the World Wide Web has become a workshop for us to learn about our ability to exchange between self and world and to create tribes, flocks, hives, pods, and other swarms of connection.

Phyllis grew up in a strict religious family that believed children should be neither seen nor heard. She was not included in discussions or decisions and was often sent off, so she didn't get to observe adults solving problems or participating in communal decision-making. When she entered her early teens, she became anorexic. In that context her eating disorder was treated as a form of "letting Satan in," so the community shunned her in an effort to force her to repudiate her "demon." Instead, she got so dangerously thin that a store owner in town reported her to the authorities, who were able to get her to a hospital and into foster care for some help.

In some ways, you could say it was clever of Phyllis's Earth Elemental Self to find a way to pull her out of that situation. But this was not just a protest nor just a psychological issue. She had a serious imbalance in her energetic equipment for bringing in and putting out energetic signals. She spent sixteen years in and out of treatment, boxing with her eating disorder in behavioral and emotional terms. The work was helpful but did not address the whole picture. Finally she made friends with a woman who was using energy medicine to heal an anxiety disorder. She realized then that the impulse to starve herself was the result of a malfunction of equipment she had never learned how to use!

I use the term "equipment" loosely. It might also be called "energy behaviors," or "mechanisms" built into your energetic makeup that allow you to work on your web of meaning and participate in the web of connections. I've discussed at length the gatekeeper, your mechanism for keeping a self. And we've explored your built-in capacity to "speak energy," and we've been dipping into the deeply sourced streams that your instrument uses to fuel your creation of self. In this chapter we'll explore some other mechanisms that play a role in your construction of self.

As I've said before, we are not freestanding units. We are part of an ongoing, dynamic energy exchange. The energies of your body are constantly moving and exchanging within you, but they are also constantly interacting with and exchanging with the larger web of connections. Working with change, healing yourself and your world, is easier if you understand how the web of connections moves and influences you, how you can work with it, and how you can participate in it in conscious and positive ways.

CONTAINERS

At first glance, you might ask: "What do containers have to do with exchange between self and world?" The short answer is that in order to exchange effectively, the *self* part of that equation has to be sturdy enough to give and receive within the *exchange* part of it.

Subtle energy forms containers in order to direct flow, to carry out functions, and to shape meaning.

I believe containers are a feature of consciousness itself. If you learn to see the swirling exchange of energies that make you up, you will notice geometric shapes that are containers, organizers for your consciousness!

Containers give boundaries and definition to an *energy set.* Think about a sentence as a container. You can take ten random words, and they don't have any synergy: *changed * born * and * the * it * forever * life * their * baby * was.* But put those words into a sentence (following the rules of syntax for sentences as containers), and they become a narrative: "The baby was born, and it changed their life forever."

This may be extremely geeky of me, but I just *love* the concept that we can create containers in order to direct flow, carry out functions, and shape meaning. Think about types of containers that give form to your existence.

You have *physical containers*, such as your skin and blood vessels and organs.

You have *mental containers*, such as your identity, your beliefs, your mental frameworks, your schedule.

You have *energetic containers*, such as your energy field (aura) and your stream pathways.

And we have another kind of container that is maybe less apparent: *inner structures* — such as bones, your sacred baton of the self, and your body weave — that organize energies from the inside out. Even though they sit at the center of the action, they give form, direct energies, and influence flow.

All energetic containers have these features:

- **They define a working unity** and hold certain energies in relationship to each other — they have syntax.
- **They shape experience** and influence the flow of energies and meaning.
- **They act as a sensor** providing information for the gatekeeper on how to maintain sanctity of self and regulate immune function.
- **They communicate with other containers** in your spectrum of consciousness.
- **They provide coherence** or glue.
- **They anchor or ground you** in time and space or whatever dimension the container inhabits.

It is interesting to notice in nature that animals create burrows, nests, territories that act as containers, protecting them and defining the parameters of their exchanges with the wider world. Of course, we do the same thing in various ways. Your gatekeeper uses containers to partition and protect your self and, of course, to keep others out.

In energetic terms, all of your containers of body, mind, and spirit influence one another. That is why if you change your belief about something, it can affect how your body's hormones move. If you create a container for your physical self — for example, buy a new home — it can shape your mental and spiritual state.

Strengthening any of your energetic containers can have a beneficial effect on the others.

∽ Play with It! ∽

Try some of these practices next time you feel chaotic and either too vulnerable or too scattered:

- **Swaddle your energies.** Swaddling will keep an infant calm by limiting her movement, so her body can regroup without added stimulation. Similarly, you can swaddle your own energies to shut down excess inputs. It is often most effective if you swaddle yourself using a gesture or even a literal cloth or blanket. (Note: don't do this while driving a car or in circumstances where you need your radar on full strength.)

  You can also swaddle a nemesis symbolically, inviting their energies to become mindful of what they are broadcasting to you and instructing your gatekeeper not to take on those broadcasts. Use this sparingly — it is always better to work with your own energies first. And it is important not to be manipulative of others. Swaddling another person should be done only with a prayer to their Wiser Self to keep them safe and to use the container you are offering as a loving gift.

- **Create geometrical shapes to serve as energetic containers.** For example, trace hearts, spirals, circles, triangles, and/or other geometric shapes on your body or around your whole self, or mentally draw shapes around a situation that you feel needs to be contained or clarified and defined.

- **Create a keyed container.** A keyed container is one that is set to resonate with a certain energy. Draw a shape and key it using one of these techniques: wear a favorite piece of clothing while creating the container, such as your lucky sweater; pick a theme song and sing it each time you trace a shape; invoke a quality using an affirmation or elemental ambassador or beloved symbol each time you interact with the container. Over time, you will be able to use the sweater, song, affirmation, or ambassador alone to reinstate your container.

- **Use symbols to contain (or give inner structure to) your energies.** Think of the power of a cross, Star of David, or lotus blossom to frame your energies.

- **Create energetically protective containers.** Set protections on a container by surrounding it with salt, smudging it with sacred smoke, calling in the sacred directions (see "Seven Sacred Gifts," page 291), surrounding a space with angels, or setting a space to resonate at the Schumann resonance of 7.83 hertz (supposedly the resonance of a healthy cell) using a laser pen at that frequency.

- **Create functional containers that help to partition energies.** Build temporary or permanent rooms or spaces in your mind, heart, or energy field that can help protect your energies and keep you safe. Some examples: use a Universal Recycling Bin to wick off unwanted energies; set up an off-site storage facility to keep things you don't want in your energy field; make a refuge of safety in your heart; or create an imaginary energetic elevator shaft to expedite the exit of lost souls from your property, placing a white light and a guardian at the door.

∽ • ∼

The container for mother earth is her atmosphere: the energetic surround that protects her from harmful rays, maintains her temperature, facilitates the movement of water, and basically keeps her whole and safe.

As our human behaviors and lifestyle choices increasingly punch holes in that container, we are experiencing just how important this protection has been. It is clear that for the earth, rapid and radical climate change is — in energetic terms — in part a container problem.

When I was a kid, one year for Christmas I got a bizarre gift from Santa: an "autograph umbrella." In case you don't know what that is, it was a white umbrella with a pen in its handle, so people could sign it. I did my best to appreciate the gift. I signed it, and I had my family sign it, and when it rained a few days later, I went out to parade with my new fashion statement — only to discover that when you autograph a white umbrella with blue ink, you get rain leaking from all the signatures and blue ink running down your face. That was the year I stopped believing in Santa Claus.

However, I do think it was one of those life lessons. If we keep scrawling our signature on mother nature, destroying the filters set up to protect us, she's going to leak all over us!

Your body also has an environment, like mother earth. It is often referred to as your *aura* or *energy field*. And, like the atmosphere around the planet, it keeps your body contained and your energies circulating and functioning. It filters what comes at you and what you put out into the web of connections.

If you trash your energy field, create holes in your protection, you will experience both the drips and runs and the overall failures of a container that is malfunctioning. This is the realm where indulging in negative behaviors — not caring for your body as a treasured partner, indulging in resentments or jealousies, allowing yourself to be constantly distracted by outside influences — can damage your ability to maintain a healthy field. Many illnesses where you feel polluted, attacked, too tight, or too loose arise from the malfunction of your energy field. So it is useful to learn some techniques for the care and feeding of your aura.

Your aura provides more than a container and barrier from the world, however. It also provides an *intelligent interface*: a filter for energies coming in and communications for energies you are sending out. Remember, subtle energies are not neutral — they are part of your consciousness constructing a self.

Play with It!

Here are some simple tools for the care and feeding of a healthy energy field. Try these and tune in to how they make you feel. Notice also how people treat you afterward:

- Establish a "smart filter" around the edge of your aura by figure-eighting along the edge between the you and the not-you. You will have to intuit or imagine where the edge is and send your eights out to reinforce it. Fill it with a color that helps to filter the energies coming into and going out of your energy field.
- Figure-eight every which way throughout your body's atmosphere to get energies moving in their healthiest manner. You can trace large, whole-body eights as well as smaller eights and even very tiny ones.
- Fill your field with a sound, like the note of a gong, to coordinate the vibration of the energies. If you do this while figure-eighting, set each eight to resonate with the sound. Similarly, you can fill your field with a color or quality.
- Spin a cut glass crystal or flip your hand back and forth throughout your aura to get the plus-minus signaling of your energies working smoothly.
- Try fluffing your field with your hands, like a pillow that has gone flat, or use gesture to sew up and repair parts that are torn.
- If you feel dead spots in your energy field, pull in extra energy from a cosmic source to juice it up.
- Use an energy screen (like the "Spinal Fluid Screen," pages 162–63) to filter out pollutants.
- Dance and move your arms around to get your energies

moving. The Celtic weave motion is particularly effective for reintegrating the weave of your energy field.

∽ • ∾

EXCHANGE WITH THE WORLD

Years ago, my partner and I (who were living in Canada at the time) visited Granada, Spain. We were touring the basement of a church, listening to explanations about its history, when I glanced at the group assembled around the guide and noticed my favorite French cousins, from Paris, standing not ten feet from me. What are the chances that I (a Jew) would run into my cousins (also Jewish) in a Catholic church, in a different country than any of us lived in, at the exact time they would be touring its basement?

A month before that, Jacob, a Czech exchange student who was staying with my mother in Michigan, took a trip to New Mexico and stopped by a spectacular bridge to admire the landscape. He realized he didn't know how to get back to his motel, so he knocked on the window of a parked car to ask directions, only to discover another of my cousins, whom he knew from Michigan, sitting with her partner and admiring the view (OK, and making out). What are the chances of that?

I'll bet you've got some stories like that as well. And studies have been done on how many degrees of separation it would take to get a letter from one random person on the East Coast to someone who knows them on the West Coast. (Not many.) We are all inter-connected energetically, and on a subtle level, communications are constantly going on that we tend to be unconscious of...until we encounter a coincidence that can't be just coincidence.

I think we are learning, though, that — like internet search engines — we have some built-in algorithms that allow us to send and receive information via the web of connections, to filter that information in support of our web of meaning, to navigate and communicate, and to receive guidance as needed.

In this context, *guidance* includes both necessary insight to support your web of meaning and help with navigating the swirling movement of energies in this entertaining web of connections we inhabit.

Built into our systems are mechanisms of exchange designed to pull information and energies in and send information and energies out. I mentioned temporary vortexes that form over problem areas (such as rips in your safety net) in chapter 12. But the permanent equipment you have for putting out and pulling in energy are the spinning, tornado-like patterns of energy called *chakras*.

A chakra is not a thing. It is a behavior of your energies, and I believe of your consciousness itself, to enable you to pull in experience, learn from it, evolve because of it, record and store it, and send out communications to the web of connections to order up similar experiences or share that learning with others.

Chakra is a Sanskrit word meaning "wheel" or "disk." The name arises from the fact that they look like spinning tornadoes or vortexes, rooted in your energetic spine and spinning out in front and back of you along your midline. Chakras can also be found spinning from palms and feet and from other places where energy exchange happens. Different healing traditions have identified different numbers and locations of chakras; in this book I have focused primarily on the seven chakras rooted along the midline, as shown in figure 13.1 (page 262).

The first time I encountered them directly, I was running my hand lightly up and down a client's midline, about two inches above her body, and I noticed that my hand kept moving vertically up and down, as if riding gusts of wind coming out of her body. They reminded me of that famous image of Marilyn Monroe, standing over a subway vent with her skirt billowing up around her. My Councils suggested I pull "guck" out of each of the vents I felt and try to equalize the pressure, so they all had more or less the same amount of wind coming out and going in.

I added "vent clearing" to my regular energy work and of course quickly learned that there is a whole massive lore around chakras. It wasn't until I studied with Donna Eden, though, that I went much deeper into these amazing energy features. And I credit her with the invitation to explore your chakras energetically and directly.

Too often in our outside-in world, information about these amazing mechanisms gets flattened down to lists of qualities and "meanings," colors and symbols, all codified into charts. I encourage you to avoid those resources for now or, if you have already learned chakra lore, to put it aside for a while. Practice encountering these instruments of exchange with the world, these tools of personal evolution, directly.

The richest interaction arises when you see chakras as doorways into your own energetic storehouses of experience. They can support you to learn, evolve, and express yourself in energetic terms. And they allow you to change not only your inner landscape but also the ways you are treated in the world.

Arelys had issues with older women. She felt both judged and unseen by her mother and grandmother. She also felt that same pattern had somehow gotten repeated in her adult life. At the time we worked together, she'd been studying with a dance teacher she revered for over four years. She complained that the teacher had never spoken to her, never called her by name, and barely seemed to look at her in class. She was trying to decide whether to cut her losses and just find a different teacher or stay and give up on needing to be noticed.

It was a chronic issue, having to do with how Arelys was treated by and interacted with the world, and also an issue that kept recurring in new forms. We decided to go for a visit to her chakras to explore how that pattern was stored.

We used a version of the protocol below, "Renovating the Rooms of Your Chakras," to investigate what templates had been installed in her chakras as gatekeeper instructions, experience, and guidance around the issue of her relationships with older women. It was a rich and insightful visit that gave Arelys lots of information about how this energy pattern had been set up. But, more significantly, Arelys called me around three days later to report that in dance class that day — her first since our work together — her teacher had interrupted herself midsentence to say, "Everyone, look at Arelys! She is doing this so well. She's such a beautiful dancer, you should learn from her example." Moreover, after class, the teacher called Arelys over and invited her to join a select dance group she was forming.

This may sound like one of those meet-the-cousins-in-Granada moments, but in fact, in the fifteen years I've been teaching this method, I've heard dozens of stories of people using this work and experiencing not just a shift within themselves but also massive shifts in how other people behaved toward them. We truly can heal ourselves *and* the world when we work with our own instruments of energy exchange.

Protocol: Renovating the Rooms of Your Chakras

Sit or lie down somewhere comfortable where you won't be interrupted. To balance myself, I like to do a few energy exercises first. You might try "Porcupine Reset" (pages 102–3) and "Anchoring in the Stabilizing Sphere" (pages 88–92), for example.

Then formulate your question or quest: some issue you want to explore via your chakras. Rather than using a yes-no question ("Am I too pushy for Mortimer?"), it should take the form of an open-ended query: "Give me insight into _____."

You can do this exploration to work with a *physical ailment* ("Give me insight into why my bladder keeps getting infected"), with *emotional issues* ("Give me insight into my defensiveness around people with new jobs"), with *spiritual issues* ("How can I deepen my connection with the Divine?"), or even with behaviors or phenomena outside yourself ("Give me insight into how I can respond more effectively to climate change").

Remember, you are looking both to gain insight and also to renovate the "rooms" (containers) of your energetic behaviors that affect your webs of connection and meaning.

1. Keeping your question in mind, choose a chakra to enter. Start with your intuition: Where is your hand drawn? Which chakra calls to you most loudly in this moment? If you are asking about a physical condition, try the chakra nearest the organs that are affected. Or if you are dealing with an emotional issue, where do you feel those emotions in your body?
2. Now, place your palm flat on that chakra for a few seconds to

connect in with it. Then, about eight inches above the surface of your body where the chakra sits, make counterclockwise circles (up on the left and down on the right) with your palm facing your body. (Note: for men, the crown chakra has a reverse flow, so men working on their crown chakra would stir clockwise to open.) Do this about eight to ten times. Stirring the energies this way opens and activates them for communication.

3. Next, imagine you are getting in an elevator, like the elevators in an underground parking garage, to go down to the first floor. Feel yourself traveling down into the chakra to the first level, and when the elevator arrives, get out and explore the room or space you find yourself in.

    If you are uncomfortable thinking of it as an underground space, then imagine the room built on the side of a hill, so you have vistas and windows and light as needed. And if you find yourself in some other kind of space altogether, go ahead and explore that space to see what it is: it will give you insights about your question and the containers related to it.

4. You have many choices once you arrive in the room. As you did when visiting the streams, explore what you find in there. See what you can notice about the room or space. Is there furniture? Are others present?

    Ask yourself, *What is going on in this space and how can I support it to become the space I need it to be?* Call on the Universal Supply Team and your Councils to help you renovate the space as needed. But make sure you are listening to what the space is telling you — better to take the time to learn from it than to just leap in to fix it, especially when you first arrive.

    If you wish, you can do some energy medicine in that room. It is especially fruitful to do a Divine hook-up: plugging one index finger into the heart of the Divine to bring in radiance and using your other hand to fill the space with radiance.

5. When you feel the space has become what it needs to be for

now, draw a five-pointed star and circle on your skin (or on the floor of the space) to help balance the elements there. Thank the space and helpers and then get in your elevator to return to the surface. Jot down anything you experienced in the room to explore later.

6. Then, get back in your elevator and descend to the second floor. Repeat the process of exploring, investigating, doing energy medicine, calling on helpers, and renovating to bring this room to the state it needs to be in for your greatest well-being. Again, when you have finished, draw the five-pointed star and circle, thank the room and helpers, and ride your elevator back to the surface. Jot down what you experienced there and return to your elevator.

7. Continue this same process, traveling down to the third through seventh floors. You may find that some levels do not need much work at all.

8. When you have finished, take the elevator back up to where you began. With your palm, close the visit by stirring clock-wise (circling up on the right, down on the left) with your palm facing your body, about eight to ten inches above the surface. (Exception: men working on their crown chakra would stir counterclockwise to close.)

9. Sit with your notes to reflect on what you have discovered. And feel into the situation you were exploring to notice if anything feels different. Then, check in periodically over the next few weeks to see what, if anything, has changed for you relative to the issue in question.

Often, one visit will take care of the problem, as we found with Arelys. With other issues, you might wish to explore each of your chakras in depth over time to see what is stored there relative to your inquiry. If you need to, you can do the seven floors in several sessions, rather than all at once.

☙ • ❧

Sometimes we don't have time to do the deep dives and concentrated visits to our chakras to really sort out what is happening with a particular issue. But they are still a wonderfully rich place to dip into for insight and guidance. I like to do the simple protocol below, "Fishing in the Chakras," at night or in the morning, when I want to see what's going on with my body, mind, or spirit around a specific concern or when I just want general guidance and conversation with my web of meaning.

Protocol: Fishing in the Chakras

When you are looking for insights, drop a line in the relevant chakra to fish for imagery, thoughts, sensations, or guidance about what might be helpful. Use your intuition to decide which chakra to "fish" or enter the chakra nearest the organ or body part related to your question. In general, the lower chakras are better for earthly issues and the upper ones better for cosmic issues. In figure 13.1 I've included a brief descriptor of my experiences with which issues are rich to explore in which chakras. But sometimes I get cosmic information from the lower chakras and earth connections from the upper ones. So usually I just let my hand choose which chakra to fish in.

1. Pose a question you would like guidance on. Use open-ended questions, such as "Give me insight into ____."
2. Choose one chakra to visit to get insight (see figure 13.1).
3. Stir the energies of that chakra with your palm facing your body, moving in counterclockwise circles (up on the left side, down on the right) about eight inches above your body. Make at least seven slow stirs. (Note: men working on the crown chakra should stir clockwise.)
4. Then cast in an imaginary fishing line, letting it sink to its own depth. As with real-life fishing, it might take a little time to get a bite.
5. Interact with what you pull up: unpack its meaning and implications, interpret it, converse with it, do energy medicine with it, connect it to a cosmic source to flood it with radiance.

6. Then either throw it back in (catch and release) or store it somewhere safe.

7. To finish, stir seven times clockwise to reset the flow. (Note: men working on the crown chakra would stir counterclockwise.)

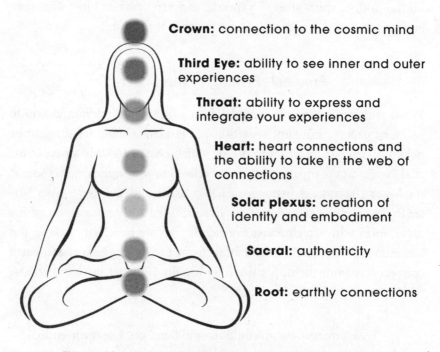

Crown: connection to the cosmic mind

Third Eye: ability to see inner and outer experiences

Throat: ability to express and integrate your experiences

Heart: heart connections and the ability to take in the web of connections

Solar plexus: creation of identity and embodiment

Sacral: authenticity

Root: earthly connections

Figure 13.1. Energetic qualities of the seven chakras

Here's an example of fishing in the chakras. I had an overly strong reaction to something someone posted on Facebook. It stuck in my craw and bothered me all day. So as I lay in bed that night, having trouble getting to sleep, I decided to go fishing to see what I could learn about the incident. My hand chose the third chakra, which I think of as my identity center. I threw in a line, and in about ten seconds, I could feel a tug. I pulled up my "catch," which turned out to be a shoebox filled with old photos. And every one of these photos was of someone who had acted as a nemesis for me — causing me problems with parents or teachers, accusing me unfairly of things I hadn't done.

For some reason, this person posting on Facebook felt unsafe to me in a similar way. I decided I didn't want to throw the box back in my chakra, didn't need to keep that rogues' gallery of people I felt harmed by. So I threw it into the Universal Recycling Bin, stirred my chakra to close it, and fell into a sound and peaceful sleep. I might decide to do a deeper dive on this issue of people who wished me ill, using "Renovating the Rooms of Your Chakras" (pages 258–60). And as for the person who had posted, I reinforced my aura by strengthening my smart filter (page 254) and invited my field to filter that person's energies out. In pragmatic terms, I decided I did not need to read her posts going forward.

POSITIVE WEBWORKING

Your energetic exchange network is something you co-create with others: friends, family, colleagues, tribe, and swarm. The task in dealing with change and cultivating well-being is to learn to make healthy webs and to transform unhealthy linkages into something more viable.

The direct and indirect exchange of energies with others creates an energetic home in this earth dimension — it provides anchors and nourishment for you. Think about how the groups you affiliate with and the beliefs you ascribe to feed you as you feel your membership accepted, shared, and enriched by other people's perceptions and experiences.

Positive webworking involves finding your tribes and strengthening the filaments of connection you share with them.

I call this personal web of connections your *spidey web*. Like spiders, we weave connections that hold us, anchor us, and provide us with a place to dwell. Some of those connections are quite temporary — think of the bond that can form in a group that experiences an amazing concert together or works intensively over several days to save people from a disaster. And some of those connections are formed and must be reinforced over time to serve as more long-term supports. Here's a practice to build and strengthen positive webworking.

Protocol: Spidey Webworking

1. Use your breath and gestures to gather yourself into your center.

2. Send individual filaments of connection to people you admire, places you love, things that inspire you.

3. Then use your hands as well as your mind to weave gifts or intentions into those web connectors. They can be nonverbal, such as a favorite color or song, or they can be verbal, such as an affirmation or prayer: "May all beings know deep peace and contentment."

   Infuse into each strand of your web whatever you wish to share in common: "I wish that we all be blessed with awakening" or "May all of us feel creature love and have balls to chase and bones to chew." I often weave these wishes horizontally among the strands I've already connected to people and places I love. Like with a spiderweb, cross-weaving can bring extra strength and support.

4. Replace strands of connection that you don't agree with between you and others with healthy, positive strands. Key them to energies you wish to be experiencing or use energy dialogue to heal the strands with color, sound, rhythm, movement. For example, if you and a family member have a soured relationship, use spidey webworking to establish some more positive filaments of connection to replace those that carry the bad blood.

A more advanced version of spidey webworking is to use this activity as a kind of vision board. If you are old enough to have attended workshops in the 1970s–1990s, you probably remember vision boards, where you'd cut pictures out of magazines representing what you wished to call into your life and paste them into an inspirational collage. In this version of spidey webworking, you create the web of connections you would like to have. Connect up with the people, places, opportunities, kinds of activities you want to see coming into your life, ones that fit your desired vision. Then infuse each strand with some of your essence, your favorite color, or the musical note that feels most comfortable to sing (your core note).

Note: Positive webworking is quite different from rooting out and removing energetic cords. I don't usually recommend this old-timey practice, because it can tear your web of meaning or web of connections in ways you can't control. Spidey webworking builds new weave and allows the old connections to simply wither away. Or you can go into your chakras to explore and transform the relationships that you feel bound into via cords.

∞ • ∞

NAVIGATION IN THE WEB OF CONNECTIONS

When I was teaching in the Eden Energy Medicine Certification Program, a colleague slipped, broke her ankle, and had to be transported to the hospital. I didn't see her again until about six months later, when we were again co-teaching. I noticed she was limping and grimacing with pain each time she stepped on one side. I asked her to fill me in on her injury.

She said, "It's the craziest thing. According to the X-rays and scans, my ankle is completely healed. It was a clean break, and the bones are now fine. And my chiropractor checked my alignment and muscles, and they are all fine, too. But it hurts like heck when I walk, you can tell it's still quite swollen compared to the other ankle, and I can't walk without limping."

I was looking at her foot as she talked and saw something I'd never seen before: a ring with colored lights streaming every which way out of the ball of her foot. My eye was drawn to her other foot, and I saw the same colored lights, but they were descending into the earth, where they met up with corresponding energies from the earth.

It looked like a sonar ring to me, an energetic communication device meant to send and receive signals from her foot to the earth.

I asked, "Can I try something?"

"Of course," she said. So I had her sit down, and I took hold of the ring I was seeing on her injured side, used her inhale to gently pull it out from where it sat, and then reseated it as she exhaled. As we sat there looking at her ankle, the swelling just disappeared, like a balloon deflating.

She stood up and said, "The pain is totally gone." She took a few steps, and she wasn't limping. And the lights I'd seen in her misaligned sonar ring were now meeting up with the lights from beneath the earth, matching her uninjured foot.

When she had injured her ankle, she knocked her sonar ring out of alignment. This caused her gatekeeper to sound the alarm about this imbalance via inflammation and pain. After I reseated the ring, her pain never returned.

I subsequently discovered there is an entire set of thirteen sonar rings distributed around the body. And over the years, I've come to understand that — like ships, and whales, and birds — we have navigational equipment. Our sonar rings allow us to navigate and to communicate with other forms and dimensions of consciousness.

Your sonar rings are receivers for and transmitters of subtle energies. They pull energies from different dimensions of consciousness into your body and translate them into the base language your body speaks. Just as our number system is base ten, your body communicates using base "element."

The sonar rings connect you with the forces of many dimensions, just as your radio connects you with different radio stations. And like a radio dial, if a ring is not quite aligned on the station, you get annoying static; when it is on the station, the sound, or sonar, flows.

Whenever you have an injury that doesn't heal fully or when your body takes a whack physically, emotionally, energetically, or spiritually, it can knock your sonars off-balance and cause static. I always check them after someone has had surgery, has been exposed to an X-ray or other scan, has had a traumatic event, has gone through an illness, or is having issues with balance.

Whenever you need support navigating your experience or feeling in touch with the swarm, it is helpful to balance your sonar rings.

Protocol: Balancing Your Sonar Rings

The thirteen sonar rings form a navigation and communication system that hooks you up with the forces of the many dimensions:

- There are twelve sonar rings on or near the body and a thirteenth large sonar ring that exists just outside your energy field.
- Each sonar ring acts as a receiver, transmitter, and translator for a particular kind of energy. It also often influences operations in the part of the body where it sits.
- The sonar rings operate both independently and as a whole system. You can use specific ones to address specific purposes.
- You can adjust the whole system to put yourself (or another person) into a more transcendent balance and equilibrium.
- Adjusting the sonar rings can help with basic energy distribution in the body (especially related to balance, grounding, and intrabody communication), as well as with more cosmic balancing.

Locations and Primary Functions

The locations and primary functions of the sonar rings are detailed in figure 13.2 and table 13.1 (see next page). Note: although each sonar ring has a primary function, they all can shift function if necessary.

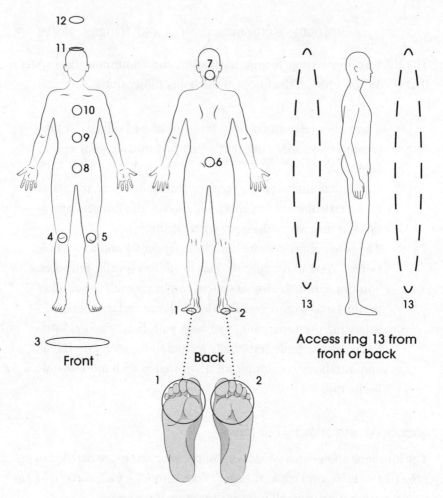

Figure 13.2. The thirteen sonar rings

Table 13.1. The locations and primary functions of the thirteen sonar rings

The Thirteen Sonar Rings		
Ring(s)	Location	Primary Function
1 and 2	**Bottoms of feet.** These rings circle the balls from the Kidney-1 points to the toe tips.	Facilitating communication with the earth elemental realm.

The Thirteen Sonar Rings *(continued)*		
Ring(s)	Location	Primary Function
3	**Fourteen inches below the feet** (earth ring). A dinner-plate-sized ring.	Reading the earth energies (earthquake activity, et cetera) and access to what is happening in other parts of the planet; communication with the planet itself as a consciousness.
4 and 5	**Knees.** These jar-lid-sized rings (four to five inches in diameter) are seated roughly around the knee cap.	Amplifying communications with the personal template. This helps with balance of personal impulse versus fulfillment (what you want versus what you can actually accomplish), including getting needs met.
6	**Ming men area on the spine.** This ring is the size of a jar lid.	Promoting flow and access to universal flows.
7	**Power point area at the base of the skull.** This ring is generally a bit smaller than the others, two and a half to three inches in diameter.	Balancing the Talking Self realm (personality, identity, sense of self) plus reading the patterns of human and extrahuman endeavors.
8	**Below the belly button (dan tien area).** This ring is about two and a half to three inches in diameter.	Establishing primal connection with all sentient beings.
9	**Solar plexus area.** This ring is the size of a jar lid.	Reading the creature realm — the entire sound spectrum can be heard here. Also provides access to the collective unconscious.
10	**Heart area.** Located in the center of the chest at the high heart, it is thicker than the others and has seven layers. Size of a jar lid.	Reading the Akashic records (the collective unconscious) — history and future and all dimensions of experience can be read here.

The Thirteen Sonar Rings *(continued)*		
Ring(s)	Location	Primary Function
11	**Top of head.** Size of a jar lid.	Reading the light spectrum and light communications.
12	**One foot above the head (sky ring).** This ring is about one foot above a person's head and can be the size of a hand grasping a jar lid or larger.	Hearing the larger symphony — communications with the other dimensions.
13	**In front and in back of the person outside the field.** The location of these two sonar rings varies, so you have to feel for them. Generally they are at arm's length plus about one foot away from the body in both front and back. Adjust only one of them. They are five to six feet in diameter, larger than the body. The best way to adjust this ring is to sing your core note, if you know it. Experiment with singing notes that make you come home to yourself energetically. Manual adjustments also work but don't last as long. Reverence can also reset it.	Connecting you with alternate realities. In *your* reality, when it is seated, it feeds the imagination and ability of the mind to travel.

Adjusting the Sonar Rings

To prepare, spoon the bottoms of your feet with a stainless-steel spoon to make sure your polarities are grounded. Use the rounded part of the spoon to rub the skin of your bare feet forward and back, side to side, and in figure-eight patterns if you wish.

Tune in to the sonar ring you want to adjust to feel if it is seated correctly or not. You can use intuition for this.

To adjust the sonar ring, inhale and pull the ring out from your body about one-quarter to one-half inch. *Do not pull the ring out any further.* You are basically grabbing the ring energetically and pulling it just free from the body. Jiggle it very gently to release it from where it was set, and as you exhale, reseat the ring by gently supporting it to go back where it belongs. It usually pulls itself back into its correct seating.

When it is reseated, hold the sonar ring in place on the body for several seconds to help fix its correct position, then trace the five-pointed star and circle on the sonar ring to rebalance its attunement to the five elements.

Once you have made the adjustment, tune in to feel if energy is now flowing more comfortably through the sonar ring and its surrounding area.

Adjusting your sonar rings can make a profound difference in how well you navigate, how balanced you feel, and how your body communicates within itself and functions in diverse situations and within the web of connections. Check your rings whenever you feel you have been knocked off-balance!

⚭ • ⚭

MIRRORING

If you studied Psychology 101 in the 1970s or '80s, you probably read the famous study on attention, where researchers asked students in several classes (unbeknownst to their teachers) to look consistently just to the right of their instructor. If the teacher shifted, they were asked to keep moving their gaze just to the right. In classroom after classroom, the teacher ended up stage right or, in some cases, offstage altogether.

We are designed to use our gaze and our attention to mirror one another.

Mirroring is having your energies received and appreciated and reflected back, feeling seen, heard, and validated.

Although the classroom experiment was a psychology study, this phenomenon of mirroring is an energetic one. In the web of connections, our energies need to feel met and responded to. If we don't receive this, our gatekeepers signal reactivity and danger to let us know we are lacking essential inputs.

In your contacts with others, any look, tone of voice, touch, or other response that you feel is inauthentic, disrespectful, distracted, critical, or unaffirming of your humanity will affect your sense of orientation and make it difficult for you to navigate the web of connections in nourishing ways.

Think about situations where you have not gotten appropriate mirroring:

- A workplace where your boss or colleagues don't acknowledge your value or you can't be seen for who you are
- A family that doesn't get your sense of humor
- A group of peers who pretend to like you but make fun of you behind your back

Any of these, or similar situations, can create chronic energetic stress and illness.

Anita got sick after her kids left home. She developed chronic fatigue, depression, and chronic ringing in her ears. Several doctors dismissed her or told her the problem was psychological. She saw a series of complementary medical practitioners, who diagnosed heavy metal poisoning, post–Lyme disease syndrome, and gut imbalance. But the treatments they offered her for these made no difference in her symptoms.

When Anita told me her story, however, the source of the problem became obvious. Anita was suffering from a mirroring issue! Her husband was polite and kind, but he had a mild version of Asperger's syndrome, a kind of high-functioning autism, and just didn't mirror her. He wasn't negative; he didn't ignore her. But when she spoke, it was like speaking to a blank wall: he had no affect, no real response. It was part of his makeup that he did not instinctively mirror others.

It was only after her kids left the nest that this became a problem. She wasn't hurt or aware of being annoyed with him. In fact, she didn't connect her issue to her husband at all, because she was used to this quirk in his makeup.

Once she realized she needed other mirroring, she made Zoom dates with relatives, volunteered to sit at the library help desk a few days a week, and planned a weekend getaway with her closest friends from college. And within about a month, she was fine.

☞ Play with It! ☜

If you have someone to help you, practice mirroring each other. Say something and ask your friend to respond in a supportive way: expressing validation with their face or their tone of voice, letting you know how your speech affected them, touching you affectionately, and so on. Then reverse roles and practice mirroring your buddy in a positive way.

You can also play games with a child or neighbor that involve sharing something back and forth. Something as simple as tossing a ball to each other and really attending to the giving and receiving, using your voice and face to celebrate the fun of the activity, can strengthen your sense of being mirrored.

When you are on your own, do your energy medicine exercises while watching yourself in the mirror. Figure-eight all over your body and between yourself and your mirror image, draw loving shapes around your body, do "Pet the Doggy / Pet the Kitty," and make other gestures of support and reciprocity. Be aware of any tendencies you might have to look at your own image with criticism or to squeeze that extra flesh on your belly — and instead practice treating yourself well, as you would a best friend, in ways you can see, hear, feel, know viscerally.

☜ • ☞

As you explore your ability to exchange in the web of connections, take a little time to think about how your connections with others have changed — because of the Covid-19 pandemic, because of shifting patterns of work and play, because of the explosion of social media. The appeal of social media is in part a response to our need for webworking and mirroring, our pull to participate in pod and swarm. But because it is a new culture, it can sometimes be like junk food — tasty but not nutritious and often habit-forming. Social media can be a lifeline, especially if you are isolated from others, but it can also be a fun house mirror that distorts your thinking and amplifies damaging groupthink.

Some of the reality show stars and social media influencers are victims of too much mirroring of the wrong sort. They get addicted to the attention, without linking it to what their soul needs to share.

And being falsely mirrored, whether by someone who does not really get you or by someone who is narcissistic or wishes you ill, can knock your sonar rings off their seating and can cause distortions in your creation of self. It can unground you, unglue you, and disrupt your flow. Use the tools in this chapter to access inner guidance on what you need. And perhaps dip into the next chapter, "Spirit in the Body," to find deeper inspiration.

⧉ Chapter Fourteen ⧉

Spirit in the Body

Shamisa was a bundle of joy. At six years of age, she glowed, which made people around her smile. But within two months of starting first grade, she was, according to Makena, her mother, a changed creature. Makena said, "Misa's not sad or depressed. It is just as if someone turned her dimmer switch to low."

Makena wasn't sure where to look for causes. Was there a physical problem? Had something terrible happened that her daughter wasn't able to articulate? That was a terrifying thought. It propelled Makena to bring Misa for an energy medicine session to get a sense of what was going on.

We decided that all three of us would send out imaginary sniffer dogs to see where the dimmer switch was. When we compared notes, all three of us saw the dogs running to Shamisa's school and into her first grade classroom.

Makena was confused by this. "She loved kindergarten and says she likes school fine." Shamisa nodded agreement but averted her gaze. She knew her mom and dad had been thrilled to have her in this particular classroom — the teacher was a thirty-year veteran with a good reputation for preparing her students academically. At the parent-teacher meeting, they had found the teacher serious and dedicated.

I taught Makena and Misa some energy medicine to support Shamisa's radiance and suggested they make sure she had some playtime each day after school to reclaim her normal rhythms.

We decided Makena would also spend a day observing her daughter's classroom. I got a call the next night. "Shamisa was her normal self when we got there, but I noticed every time she moved, the teacher directed her to concentrate. And when Misa giggled while answering a question, the teacher didn't smile but instead asked her to repeat her answer and try to stay focused."

It was clear to Makena that the teacher had set out to teach her daughter focus and discipline but was instead tamping down Misa's natural ebullience and teaching her to dim her light. Makena and her husband had already spoken to the principal about getting Misa moved to another classroom with a younger, more playful teacher who would be a better fit. Luckily, they had options. I've had many clients face much more agonizing choices in trying to safeguard their children's radiance!

Chances are, you've also faced some tough choices in trying to safeguard yours. *Radiance* is the sixth aspect of cultivating well-being and working with change. Radiance is the energy of your spirit: your soul juice, mojo, whatever makes you feel fully alive. Your radiance fuels you to navigate change and empowers you to transform from the inside out.

I used to call it the "glee factor" in young kids. It is a latent ability, like our potential for learning a language, that needs to be actively developed through interaction and support for your individual spirit and nature.

As young children, we are born with the capacity for radiance and delight. But we need to learn the care and feeding of our radiance — how to cultivate it and how to activate it in our mind and body. We need support (including positive mirroring) in learning true enjoyment.

Shamisa had glee factor in spades; it was natural to her, because she had a lot of fire element in her. And she was one of those lucky children who awakened response in the people around her. She was naturally expressive, outgoing, and attuned to other people. So in her first six years her spirit came forth into everything she did... until she encountered a teacher who refused to mirror her sparkle and set about trying to teach Misa's gatekeeper to be more low-key, measured, disciplined, and sedate — a real violation of Misa's natural instrument.

Your radiance is the cosmic partner of your gatekeeper. It acts as a resource and guardian of your soul's truth.

Radiance is your source qi, the animating, expanding, expressive force. The gatekeeper is your shaping, containing, and protective force.

We need both. But once in a while we encounter someone, like Shamisa's teacher, whose own gatekeeper constrains our radiance to such an extent that it dims or is no longer accessible to fuel our body and spirit.

In an ideal world, our gatekeepers are shaped from the inside out. They are softened, enlivened, consoled, and inspired by our own radiant spirit. In our less-than-ideal world, you may benefit from learning ways to cultivate spirit in your body and reclaim your radiance!

HOW RADIANT ARE YOU?

Here are some questions for you. On a scale of 0 to 100, what is your glee factor? How much enjoyment are you able to derive from life? How alive do you feel?

Radiance is not just high energy; it is your unique soul energy expressing itself through your body and mind. Radiance is also not just animation or joy; it is activation of that X factor in you that makes you most fully *you*. Embodying your spirit takes different forms in different people.

∽ Play with It! ∽

Radiance Self-Assessment Guide

Think of a moment or moments when you have felt *fully alive.*

1. What are five words you would use to describe that feeling?
2. How do you access your own radiance, sense of being alive, soul juice?

3. What supports you to feel fully alive?
4. What keeps you or blocks you from being fully alive right now?
5. In what ways does your body express your spirit and embody it?
6. How often during the week do you consciously access or cultivate your own radiance?

Radiance and the Five Elements

What form(s) does radiance take for you? To get a sense of how much radiance you experience in a typical week, rate your experience of each of the following types of radiance on a scale of 0 to 10, where 0 is never, 5 is occasionally, and 10 is frequently. This will give you a profile of the types and extent of radiance moving in your life:

- **Water radiance** may feel like a pervasive sense of well-being, or you may appear to glow or be illuminated from within. You feel deeply moved, motivated from inner knowing.

    How it moves: wonder and a sense of being and flow.
- **Wood radiance** may appear to be joyous and triumphant, inspiring and thrilling. You are focused on what can be built or aspired to.

    How it moves: growing, planning and designing, marching with purpose.
- **Fire radiance** may be a sparkly, celebratory kind of joy or excitement. You may appear to be on fire with inspiration and creativity.

    How it moves: celebrating, illuminating, skipping or jumping for joy.
- **Earth radiance** may be expressed as contentment and satisfaction, a sense of maternal pride and support for all. You radiate mother love and compassion.

    How it moves: nurturing, comforting, meandering.
- **Metal radiance** can be a kind of resonance and awareness.

You may feel a quiet sense of purpose and of being on the right path, a clarity of seeing or knowing.

How it moves: organizing or structuring, evaluating, distilling, proceeding in royal fashion, or staying still.

∽ • ∾

CULTIVATING RADIANCE

Certain activities bring me alive but totally drain my partner and vice versa. I love to grocery shop; she wilts or gets impatient. She loves to iron and vacuum, both of which exhaust me. But we both are enlivened by travel, even a dorky outing to a gluten-free bakery!

Whatever brings you alive is part of your vibrational nutrition — your energy diet. And when you can cultivate the energies that feed you through your everyday life, you are more likely to keep your radiance humming and feel a sense of being alive.

Although each of us has access to the cosmic qi of the streams, we also each have very individualized sources of radiance I call *spirit feeds*. These are cosmic energies that support specific themes or roles in your life. For example, I'm a messenger. I'm a teacher/traveler. I'm a framer. I'm a storyteller. I'm a healer. These roles are reflective of cosmic energies that make me feel alive whenever I'm using them.

Take a moment to explore what most enlivens you. It is great to then figure out what the energetic nature of that activity is. For example, if you love ironing, chances are you love the smoothing of wrinkles, the transformation from messy to neat, or the fire and metal combination of the iron. And if you love collecting old farm tools, perhaps you love either cultivation of the earth, or celebrating history, or the pragmatics of fitting tools to a specific task.

Whatever objects, activities, or focus most bring you alive, they are an indication of your spirit feeds, and they will nourish you most fully in your energy diet. Similarly, activities that kill your radiance, exhaust you, or make you feel dead inside are ones to weed out of your repertoire, as best you can. I'll be honest, I rarely iron or vacuum anymore!

What truly fuels you? If you're a windmill, you need wind. If you're a waterwheel, you need water. If you're a gas engine, you need gas. Putting gas into a windmill is not going to fuel you.

The goal of cultivating radiance is to construct a life where you can tap into the energies that most feed you in as many forms as possible within your everyday existence.

OPENING THE DOORS TO RADIANCE

Lots of your energy equipment can be used to open the doors to radiance. For example, adjusting your sonar rings will help you access cosmic energies that will fuel you as well as helping you navigate. Unclogging your chakras or strengthening your body weave are also excellent ways to help your body take in and use radiance. Clearing your energy streams and tapping into their cosmic sources can do the trick.

"Open Sesame" (pages 108–10) can support your gatekeeper to let radiance in. And the following protocol, "Opening Your Cosmic Gates," is one of my go-to choices whenever I notice my radiance is low.

Protocol: Opening Your Cosmic Gates

The cosmic gates are the doorways between you and all possibility.

The First Cosmic Gate

The first cosmic gate sits at approximately arm's length plus one foot in front of you (see figure 14.1). It is large, extending about a foot above and below the outline of your body. (Note: it is not the same as the thirteenth sonar ring but sits quite near it.)

When some part of your being feels cosmically challenged (in a negative or positive way), your cosmic gate may swing shut and latch or even lock. If you don't unlock it, unhook the latch, and open the gate, you are likely to experience recurring disarray in your body and mind, and you'll have trouble accessing the guidance of your spirit. You can use your intuition to feel if a cosmic gate has swung shut and is locked. Extend your

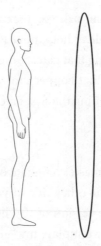

Figure 14.1. First cosmic gate

hand, palm facing the gate, and feel into whether it is locked. (If you know energy testing, it should test strong with your palm facing the gate and weak if facing away — a polarity test. If it doesn't, it needs correction. See appendix A.) But don't worry if you can't feel its status. Unlocking an unlocked gate doesn't lock it!

To unlock the cosmic gate, reach out with both hands and use gesture to grab it by the top and bottom. Flip the gate vertically so the outer side faces in and the inner side faces out.

To open the latch, reach out to make contact with the latch energetically and unlatch it. I usually picture a hotel room hasp lock (see figure 14.2) and flip it open with my finger. You can also turn a door handle if that's how you picture it. Inhale, then on the exhale unlatch it.

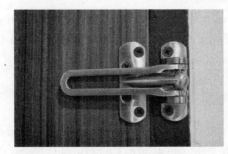

Figure 14.2. Latch

Now, imagine placing your palm on the cosmic gate and gently push it open, again using your exhale to help move the energy. You may encounter some resistance to opening that gate. Sometimes we just aren't ready to face our larger potential! If that happens for you, do "Open Sesame" first (pages 108–10), then try opening the first gate.

The Harmonic Self

Your harmonic self is like a master template or blueprint that guides your gatekeeper. She stands on the other side of your first cosmic gate, opposite your embodied self (the version of you here in body; see figure 14.3). I sometimes call this master template my "always self," because she represents what I think is generally true about me, even when it isn't obvious. For example, I believe I've got great lungs. This truth is coded into my harmonic self (my always self) so that even on the rare occasion that I get a cold in my lungs, this infirmity is not reflected in my harmonic self if I energy test her lungs.

This master template, your harmonic self, is co-created by you, based on your own experiences and beliefs, and your Wiser Self. So it is a great place to visit to work on changing beliefs and habits that seem to be part of who you believe yourself to be or how your body "always" seems to react.

You can figure-eight between your body and your harmonic self and do energy medicine on your harmonic self to influence your body and shift habits. For example, you can take her out of porcupine reactivity, or draw hearts on her heart, or anchor her in a stabilizing sphere. To do this, you will have to mime the actions, projecting them onto her, since she stands beyond arm's reach.

Your harmonic self is a rich place to do energy medicine, because sometimes your energy challenges don't reside in your body; they emanate from this master template!

The Second Cosmic Gate

If your harmonic self turns and faces away from you and extends her arm, the second cosmic gate sits at arm's length plus about one foot beyond your harmonic self (see figure 14.3).

First cosmic gate   Second cosmic gate

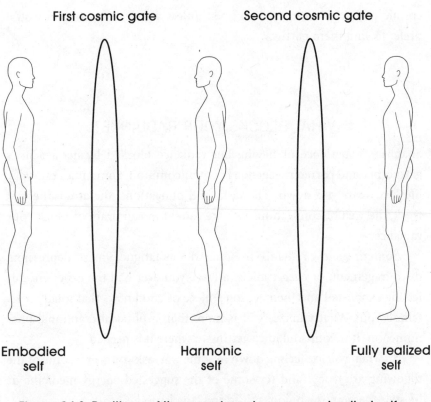

Embodied   Harmonic   Fully realized
self   self   self

Figure 14.3. Positions of the cosmic gates, your embodied self,
harmonic self, and fully realized self

You can feel with your outstretched palm (or use an energy test, as mentioned above) to see if that second cosmic gate is locked. If it is, unlock it by flipping the whole gate from bottom to top, using your exhale, so the front faces the back. Now, reach out or have your harmonic self reach out and use gesture to unlatch the latch. Inhale and, on the exhale, gently push open the second gate.

Your Fully Realized Self

On the other side of the second gate you will find your fully realized self. This is a wonderful source of guidance and coherence. Figure-eight between your fully realized self and your harmonic self, then between your harmonic self and your embodied self. Tune in to how you feel with your cosmic gates open. Leave them open unless you feel unsafe and would prefer to shut them partway.

∽ • ∽

WHAT BLOCKS YOUR RADIANCE?

Shamisa's experience of having her radiance blocked by her teacher's gatekeeper and corrective agenda is not uncommon. Sometimes everyday life just wears you down. The tasks and obligations, the atmosphere at work, the web of connections you are caught in can drain or block your radiance.

Sometimes low radiance masquerades as fatigue, illness, depression, discouragement, or even cynicism. Have you ever had the experience of feeling exhausted and then getting a piece of good news that totally revitalized you? What vitalizes you is more than a physical-emotional phenomenon. It is your soul juice getting to where it is needed.

So when you are feeling down in some way, ask yourself if some of the following are true...and try some of the suggested energy medicine or lifestyle medicine techniques to address the issue.

∽ Play with It! ∽

1. **I have a low glee factor.** Imagine you are an infant again, freshly discovering your world, and go into sensory motor explorations. Let yourself turn off your thoughts and just encounter tastes, sounds, feels, smells, and visuals around you. Get yourself into an environment that generally nourishes you: in the woods, beside a stream, in a garden, on a mountain, or even in a sanctuary room you've set up in your heart or house for this purpose.

    You can reinforce your body weave (pages 201–3) or do a "Harmonizing Hook-Up" (page 237), "Open Sesame" (pages 108–10), or any of the exercises in this chapter. Make a habit of asking yourself with each activity of your day: *How can I bring radiance into what I am doing? How can I make this enjoyable or fulfilling?*

2. **I never learned to find my radiance.** As mentioned just above, let yourself enjoy playing with sensory motor explorations. Take some time to brainstorm, alone or with a friend, about what some of your spirit feeds might be.

   Open your cosmic gates (pages 280–84). Do the twelve hearts exercise: draw three hearts over your head, three hearts over your torso, three hearts over your pelvic bowl, and three hearts over your entire body. Adjust your sonar rings (pages 267–71) and strengthen your body weave (pages 201–3).

3. **I confuse radiance (illumination from within) with excitement or stimulation (animation from without).** Anchor yourself in a stabilizing sphere (pages 88–92), strengthen your body weave (pages 201–3), and go through the "Radiance Self-Assessment Guide" (pages 277–79) to see what forms your radiance naturally takes.

4. **I don't know who I am, what kind of energetic fuel I need.** Open your cosmic gates (pages 280–84), do the "Harmonizing Hook-Up" (page 237), work on your gatekeeper. And visit your streams — particularly heart/connection (pages 138–39), yin protector (pages 134–36), and your earth streams (pages 170–76) — to ask the questions: *Who am I, and what do I need to do in order to nourish my spirit?*

5. **I am too broken, sick, tired, discouraged, depressed, et cetera.** Reinforce your body weave (pages 201–3) and clear your sacred baton of the self (pages 154–56). Visit the streams, one a day, for fourteen days. Let your body show you the way to inner radiance.

CO • ⊙

SPIRITUAL WISDOM

In the context of working from the inside out, spiritual wisdom might also be described as "seeing with the eyes of radiance." It is about how to tap into your own sources of wisdom and guidance via your body. From that perspective, radiance brings you clarity on who you are and how you can best navigate life.

The outside-in version of spiritual wisdom is tempting: having a psychic tell us who we are, letting a guru instruct us on how to live, reading expertise from lifelong spiritual seekers who now have recipes for you to follow. And there is value in some of these, within reason.

However, I have had so many clients say to me, "I've been told …" and then quote some expert who implanted some truth that just doesn't look true from *my* outside-in viewpoint. And I've tried so many methods from people who directed me on what to do, but not on how to figure out what my truth was.

So I think your best bet is to invest time in activating your built-in equipment for knowing and befriending your own consciousness, in order to discover your unique truth from the inside out.

Here's an exercise my Councils gave me to activate my inner knowing.

Exercise: Expand to Your True Size

Choose a place to do this where you feel safe and comfortable, preferably alone, or at a time when you don't expect interruptions. This is best done in bed, or in an easy chair, or outside in a protected area.

Start by Celtic-weaving your aura (weaving both hands in and out in figure-eight patterns, crossing at the center). Then place both palms on your midline to center yourself.

Take a few moments to breathe in and out, feeling your breath enter and leave. With each inhale, gather your energies in. With each exhale, release any tensions or preoccupations.

Then, when you are ready, allow yourself to expand to your true size, perhaps using your exhales to expand your everyday boundaries outward. Hint: your true size is probably larger than the planet.

Once in that state, just inhabit it, experience it. Stay in it for as long as you wish.

When you are ready, return to your everyday size, following your breath in and out and touching your body to remember the boundaries of this embodied self.

☯ • ☯

The kind of insight you can get from this type of activity is something I call *field knowing*. You are knowing the feel of a different energy state — a field. That is so different from learning some abstract concepts about reality or spiritual truth from different traditions and then trying to apply them to your life. Many meditation techniques and yoga techniques can support your field knowing.

In a nutshell, I believe that the more wisdom you can get from the embodiment of your spirit and the guidance of your soul, the better off you are. Sometimes someone else's truth will really set a gong resonating for me. It'll activate my own knowing. But if I don't already have some of that knowing in myself, it's just a memorized thing that I go on to spout to others. I may sound wise, but it is not really wisdom that supports my ability to navigate and evolve in alignment with my soul.

LARGER MIND, SMALLER MIND

Years ago, my Councils told me, "We have a concept to teach you. It's called *larger mind, smaller mind.*" They said, "Imagine that we pick you up and put you into a very large bowl of floating island."

Now, if you are thinking, "Oh, *île flottante*, that delicious French dessert," that's not what they meant. They were referring to a dessert my mother found in a women's magazine in the 1950s, which was essentially a large bowl of vanilla pudding with a can of fruit cocktail stirred into it. They continued:

> If you find yourself in that large bowl of floating island, it might take you a while to figure out where you are. You'll maybe taste the white stuff and say, "Hmm, vanilla pudding." And you'll maybe

swim a bit and encounter an odd orange cube and realize it's a chunk of peach. And you keep swimming and keep needing to figure out what all you are encountering. That's smaller mind.

And then, if you keep swimming, at some point you notice you now have a sense of how much fruit is in the bowl, and where the sides of the bowl are, and maybe how to chart a course from the second pear chunk to the maraschino cherry near the bottom of the bowl. Once you can map your progress, maybe even find shortcuts, you are in larger mind. That's how you evolve and learn and grow.

Smaller mind is another name for beginner's mind. In the initial moments of encounter with a situation, you are in smaller mind. You are in a purely sensory motor state, taking in information, encountering each moment and each event on its own terms. You do not have maps yet, so you have to just stay present and learn. This can be sensually fulfilling and exciting — or overwhelming if you are uncomfortable without a clear sense of control.

At some point, when you have enough experience and exploration, you shift into larger mind. In this state, the parts are all encoded into your experience, and you can now create maps of how the parts relate to the whole. In larger mind you can navigate strategically, plotting shortcuts and seeing the larger picture.

It is useful to know when you are in smaller mind and when you are capable of larger mind and to embrace each of these states on its own terms. It is equally useful to recognize when you are in transition from one to the other: gaining the ability to plot a course but still lacking the full larger mind perspective to make good maps or, conversely, feeling ready to graduate from your experience and expertise to launch into new territory and experience smaller mind again.

We go from smaller mind to larger mind and back to smaller mind again and again in life as we encounter different situations. Say you're well established in a job, at the top of your game, familiar with everyone you work with and all the procedures — in larger mind. Then, one day, you are offered a promotion, and as you step into your new role you discover you are back in smaller mind, needing to open to the journey of discovery once again.

We have different tasks and competencies in smaller mind and larger mind. So it's helpful to stop and ask: *Where am I relative to this decision or choice, relative to this relationship or situation? In smaller mind? In larger mind? Or somewhere in transition between the two?*

Skillful navigation is a huge part of spiritual wisdom: skillfully navigating your life; skillfully navigating really scary, overwhelming experiences, including health challenges; skillfully navigating not knowing, being lost, being back in the pudding.

One of the important aspects of spiritual navigation is timing. What might work for you today could be a technique you had tried last year with no success. What will transform your world may not do so *now*, if your evolving self has chosen some smaller mind experiences it needs before it can emerge on the other side of the bowl.

This is particularly relevant when you are seeking guidance within and trying to make decisions. Sometimes the guidance you get is where you need to swim and explore next, not the way to get to the final destination. And that is appropriate. Too often we want to know what the right decision is, the best choice for all time, and yet we may not yet be at the choice point.

This is awkward if the choice you need to make involves time-limited opportunities. But the fact is, if you aren't at the choice point for that opportunity, it will not serve you, however tempting it sounds. The same is true of the *healing moment*. Some health challenges will resolve as a result of the journey, but not now, if you are still in smaller mind and needing to learn what the challenge is flagging for your attention.

Sometimes, when you submit to smaller mind, larger mind will rise up and lift you right out of it. It's a little like sailing. If I want to get from here to there, I can't usually go in a straight line. I have to tack back and forth and use the winds as they're moving today. Tomorrow I might have to take a different path to get to that same place on the other shore.

Take what you know about sailing. Take what you know from your own experience about larger mind and smaller mind and bring it to bear when you approach self-healing and change.

GUIDANCE

Your body is a veritable treasure chest of guidance if you are willing to enter your energies and participate in the conversations available to you there. Your Wiser Self guides you through every aspect of your body and mind, far beyond the cues you hear in your head. Your Councils echo through your instrument with insights, knowing, recognitions, awakening, and more.

Most of the methods I've taught in this book will help you not only balance your energies but also learn from them. Below are two more exercises that are particularly useful for letting your inner wisdom teach you over time, perhaps with a larger curriculum than you would dream up on your own.

Exercise: One Hundred Gifts of the Heart

Place both hands over your heart and get centered, breathing in and out, watching your breath and feeling it enter and leave. Then, ask your heart for one gift. Accept whatever comes to mind without judging it or bargaining for something better. Thank your heart for the gift and then, over the next day or two, unpack the significance and potential of that gift for you. If you don't immediately understand, just stay open to learning, getting new insight, having experiences that show you what that gift can be for you. The gifts might be quite ordinary — butter, a letter opener — or may be more cosmic in nature.

When you are ready after a day or two, repeat the process above and receive another gift. Let this process be a practice you do over several months, until you have received one hundred gifts from your heart! Make sure to track the gifts and your insights and experiences in your Book of Shadows. Your heart has the power to take you on unexpected journeys, one gift at a time!

∽ • ∾

Exercise: Seven Sacred Gifts

The seven sacred gifts in this exercise will come from and be given to the seven directions used in most earth-based sacred traditions: in front of you, behind you, to the left of you, to the right of you, above you, below you, and within you. You will be circling with your palm facing each direction in turn.

First, *in front of you*, palm facing forward, circle with your hand in a clockwise direction (up on the left and down on the right). Do this for seven to twelve rotations, until you feel done. Give a gift from your heart to that direction.

Then circle your palm counterclockwise for seven to twelve rotations. Request a gift from that sacred direction.

Next, *behind you*, do the same: circle first clockwise and give a gift, then circle counterclockwise and receive a gift.

Proceed through the rest of the directions, each time with your palm facing in that direction: *in front of you, behind you, to the left of you, to the right of you, above you, below you*, and then *within*. For each direction, circle clockwise and give a gift, then circle counterclockwise and receive a gift. For within, it usually feels good to make circles on the chest around the heart.

By doing this, you are aligning yourself with each sacred direction and reestablishing your harmony with the universe. It resets your energies for a balanced give-and-take with the world.

Notice or jot down the gifts you receive. You can interpret them later, in relation to the direction: ahead is where you are headed; behind is where you have been; the left is your receptive, yin side; the right is your more active, yang side. Above is your sky feed, the cosmic energies. Below is your earth feed, the embodiment energies. And within is the contribution of your own inner truth and heart.

☙ • ❧

YOUR PASSAGE HOME TO SOURCE

Sometimes I feel like my belly button has a lot of energy stored in it. Experiment with yours. What happens if you put a finger in it (or on it, if it's an outie) and pull it up, down, left, right, and at various angles? What do you feel in your body?

When you are in the womb, your umbilicus is your connection to Mom: you get your oxygen, food, and link with this world through it. And when you are born, that conduit is cut, literally and figuratively, and you need to learn to breathe on your own and, over time, to nourish yourself from the fruits of mother earth. Your umbilicus is a crucial link to the world you are born into.

According to my Councils, we have another umbilicus — an energetic one. It anchors at the surface of your body in the ming men area of the spine, on the back behind the belly button, and then travels inward, making a connection home to the world we are born from: our source.

Called the *ming men passage*, this is a sacred space that is helpful to visit and, if needed, to reinstate. It is important to keep that passage home open and available to the embodied soul that you are. Like opening the cosmic gates, clearing the ming men passage improves your access to your inner wisdom and Wiser Self.

Protocol: The Ming Men Passage

Like all sacred journeys, visits to the ming men passage need to be carried out in safe circumstances, in a secure place where you can do this exploration without distractions. It can be done sitting, lying down, or even standing, whichever is most comfortable. I often set a time limit on my visit to the ming men passage, especially if I decide I am going to follow the passage home. You can set an alarm or ask a friend to act as timekeeper and midwife.

Do some preliminary exercises to balance your energies: the "Porcupine Reset" (pages 102–3) and "Anchoring in the Stabilizing Sphere" (pages 88–92), for example. Then:

1. Reach around to your back and place your hand on your ming men area (on your spine opposite your belly button,

around the L2, L3, and L4 vertebrae, between your kidneys). If you can't reach it, lie on something, such as a stuffed sock, that puts a light pressure on the area.

2. Take several deep breaths while holding this spot.

3. Then, if you wish, release the hold, but sink your attention down through the ming men into the passage behind it (inside of you). You may find yourself in a kind of tube or tunnel attached at that spot, or you may find yourself in some kind of open space. If you can't find the passageway, ask the Universal Supply Team to install one and anchor it at your ming men area.

   If you find a passageway but it is disturbed, torn, clogged, or otherwise disrupted, take some time, with the help of the Universal Supply Team, to reinstate it so it can serve as a healthy inner passage for you.

4. When your passage can be traveled, follow it along to the other end, wherever that leads you. It is meant to arrive at the entrance to your passage home. The entrance might be a bridge, a tunnel, a doorway. Just look for where it is supposed to lead (it does not always correspond to a physical location in your body) and ask for help from the Universal Supply Team to get it attached at the inner end to your passage home.

5. Once you are satisfied that the ming men passage is fully reinstated, you can stop your journey there and return back to the ming men area of your spine, or you can continue to explore, crossing the bridge or entering the passage home.

   Before you continue, pause and remind yourself of one thing you want to stay in this life for: a loved one, a pet, to see a place you yearn to visit, or anything else that has meaning for you. Doing this sets a marker to facilitate the journey back into your body consciousness.

6. If you cross the bridge / pass through the tunnel / go through the doorway, ask your Councils to meet you on the other side. This is a sacred visit home, and it is not meant to be a leap into other worlds. Instead, stay in the area of where the

passage anchors within you and meet up with your Councils and Wiser Self for guidance, conversation, or just the joy of a visit home.

7. Then thank the parts of yourself you have met there and re-turn back across the bridge or through the tunnel or doorway. Travel back along the ming men passage to your energetic spine. If you wish, place your hand again on your ming men area. Take at least three deep breaths to bring your attention fully back into your earth elemental home.

�∽ • ∽

Radiance (and the wisdom it brings you) is the gift of your own spirit animating this life. It illuminates your experience with meaning, brings your gatekeeper into balance, helps you to center and ground, root and anchor. It provides coherence to your choices and flow to your under-standing and actions. It is the force that attracts the highest and best kind of exchanges to you in the web of connections.

Taken together, the six dynamics of well-being — *gatekeeping, ground-ing, coherence, flow, exchange between self and world,* and *radiance* — will change your world...and the world you co-create with all of humanity.

⤳ Conclusion ⤳

Let Your Body Show You the Way!

As I rounded the corner to finish this book, after taking two months off to help my mother in her final days, I completely ran out of steam. I felt exhausted, drained, emotionally wrecked, and as if I had crashed my adrenals and thyroid. I wasn't sure if what I was feeling was emotional, mental, physical, metabolic, spiritual, or all of the above.

Tuning in, I called up a sniffer dog and asked her to show me where the crash was coming from. She trotted down to my intestines and looked at me, wagging her tail as if to say, "Where's my treat?"

I traveled down into my gut. What I saw there looked like a road roller had run through, flattening the flora and fauna meant to be growing in my gut: my microbiome. It was as if something had tamped down the microorganisms' outreach and growth, draining them of their soul juice.

So I connected in with them using one hand, and with the other, I sent my energetic reach into some rich organic soil, to link up with a healthy biome there. I invited my little gut beasties to commune with and entrain with the mother lode. I could feel the energies of the healthy organisms communicating with and revitalizing my gut, reminding my microswarm of what health and well-being and a functioning community looked like.

I checked in hourly and repeated the hook-up entrainment, and within a day my gut was flourishing and my symptoms were gone. To keep them gone, I added in some gut-healthy foods, knocked off sugar, and increased the activities that feed me, including some serious cat-petting time. I took time to celebrate my mother's life. And I kept in touch with my gut several times a day, making sure the swarm inside me was getting what it needed to flourish. I visited my choice/discernment (small intestine) stream and my distiller/refiner (large intestine) stream to do some cleanup. And I did my best to release the stressors that were wiping out my microbiome.

Energy medicine offers you lots of tools to help you to heal, to build resilience, and to go beyond merely healing illness. It allows you to really inhabit your body, mind, and spirit as a full participant in creating your life and co-creating the world. It is full of activities to support you in living from the inside out and in reinventing our shared reality.

And from my perspective, our shared reality *needs* us to participate and reinvent the world to be a place generated from within and enlivened by spirit. Our earth needs us.

Your body is your receiver and your home office for the communications array that is your body, mind, and spirit. So starting with your body and letting it show you the way is, in my experience, a wonderful and reliable place to launch from.

If you've made it through the multiple concepts and activities I've shared from my Councils' training and my own experiences with self-healing and client support, I congratulate you. I've offered a lot of material for you to play with, and I hope you will take it in that spirit and make it yours.

But if, at this point, you are still trying to sort out all this information and figure out your own take, here's my recommendation: Keep it simple. Go inward and let your internal guidance show you. Work with these six aspects of constructing a self: *gatekeeping, grounding, coherence, flow, exchange between self and world,* and *radiance.* They will help you weave a rich energetic tapestry that gives you the resilience to initiate, navigate, and flourish within change.

Here is a recap of some of the strategies offered in this book:

1. **Show up for yourself.** Put aside your need to know what is wrong and instead assess what is needed *in this moment*. Recognize when you are capable of being in larger mind versus needing to be in smaller mind and just ask what can be done in this moment, in this place.

2. **Ask better questions.** Instead of looking for what is wrong, you are looking for what might be *right*, right now. And you are looking for what your body wants you to know right now.

3. **Recognize the role of each self.** If your mind is trying to dominate, take the time to listen to your Earth Elemental Self and make space for Wiser Self to shift your perspective. Explore reframes to liberate your mind from being stuck on old diagnosis and treatment models. Respect pain as a message from all three selves and enter the pain to travel to the other side of it.

4. **Recognize that you are co-creating a self, a life, a world.** Ask yourself what you want to contribute to your creation of self, life, and world in this moment that is viable.

5. **Let your heart give you gifts.** Wisdom can come in small ways that accumulate, like puzzle pieces. It can also come by igniting a light in your heart and mind!

6. **Get guidance from different parts of your self.** Ask your three "brains" — heart, gut, and head — to weigh in. Also use the body's own language to let it show you what it wants you to see: both symbolic language and touch, color and light, sound and rhythm, movement and gesture, smell and taste, and direct knowing. Be satisfied with insight into what you need *now*, what the next step is. When you try to encompass larger mind without the experience of smaller mind, you are likely to embrace other people's understandings and solutions rather than finding your own!

7. **Go fishing.** Cultivate a sense of being willing to wait for the fish to show up, being present on the journey rather than in a hurry to get to the destination. Send sniffer dogs to find the focal point for right now. Let your hands show you the

way. Explore whether your camel is carrying too many straws and what you can do to clear the camel's back. Drop into the streams to learn what is needed or to influence the energies that govern your body's function. Ask yourself whether there are templates of earlier experiences co-creating your present challenge and, if so, clear the templates. Open your cosmic gates and reset your sonar rings to allow for clearer navigation and communication. Interact with yourself as a beloved rather than a recalcitrant child or stubborn beast of burden.

8. **Entrain to positive teachers.** Find out where the energies live that you want to connect with and let your energies learn from them.

9. **Ask yourself which energy dynamics are front and center for you right now:**

    •   Is your **gatekeeper** communicating and needing help with *safety, identity, clearing templates / shifting habits, distribution*?

    •   Do you need **grounding,** including *release, rooting/nourishment, centering,* or *anchoring*?

    •   Where is your glue or **coherence**? Do you have enough glue to hold things together? What needs do you have for *purpose / guiding vision, connectors, structure, integration/synchronization*?

    •   What is happening to help your energies **flow** the way they are designed to flow? Are you able to *source qi, distribute it, sustain healthy circulation, influence your qi*?

    •   How is your **exchange with the world**, present and past, affecting you now? Do you have *adequate containers, healthy exchange, positive webworking,* and *healthy mirroring*?

    •   Do you need to activate your **radiance**? Can you activate your own personal radiance? Where are you in perspective (larger mind or smaller mind)? Where are you turning for guidance? Can you see with the eyes of spirit (and of Earth Elemental Self and of Talking Self) and let them collaborate? Do you have adequate abilities to *cultivate radiance, integrate spirit into body and mind, access spiritual wisdom (see with the eyes of radiance)*, and *tap into radiant guidance*?

10.   **Give yourself permission to interpret your experience from the inside out.** Remember that your body knows how to heal and to adapt to change and that your job is to support it to do that. Remember that healing is first and foremost a *communication* task. Tune in to what and how you are communicating and make more conscious choices about what kind of relationship you want with your body, mind, and spirit.

Listen. Perceive. *Have fun*, be playful. Let your body show you the way!

∾ Appendix A ∾

Simple Energy Self-Test

Although my emphasis in this book is on tuning in to perceive energies directly, it is useful to develop some skill with energy testing as well.

1. This Eden Energy Medicine energy self-test works on the pendulum principle. Stand up with both feet together, tuck each elbow into your side, and place your hands together on your solar plexus, one over the other (see figure A.1).

2. Sway a bit forward and back, just to feel your balance loosen. Then say something you know to be true: "My name is [Ellen]." Release your standing balance and allow your body to sway backward or forward in response to that statement.

3. Normally, the body sways forward or toward the truth (your yes), and it sways backward or away from something untrue (your no). Occasionally I meet someone for whom this pattern is reversed. If you massage your K-27 points (see page 224) you can often reset your pattern, so you fall forward for yes. Otherwise, just work with the pattern that presents itself.

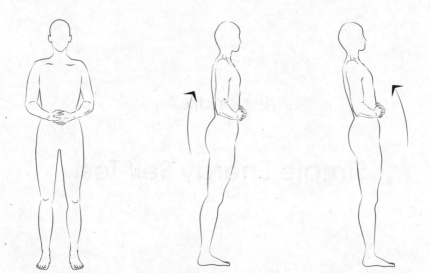

Starting position   **Fall forward for "yes"**   **Fall backward for "no"**
                              or strong energy flow   **or weak energy flow**

Figure A.1. Pendulum self-test

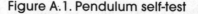

4. Try a phrase you know to be untrue: "My name is Merga-troyd." Release your standing balance and see which way your body sways.

5. Once you have calibrated this pendulum self-test to reliably sway in one direction when you state energetic truths and in the opposite direction for untruths, you can use it to validate your body-based intuition.

6. To use the pendulum self-test to energy test your halos (see pages 104–6), stand up with both feet together, tuck one elbow into your side, and place that hand on your solar plexus.

7. With your other hand, you will *energy localize* each halo. To energy localize your main halo, put your hand eight inches above your head, as if it is resting on the halo, with your palm facing your body. Let your body sway forward or back, as described above. Then flip your hand on the halo, so the palm is now facing away from your body (toward the sky), and repeat

the sway test. If you get a strong test (swaying forward) with the palm facing the body and a weak test (swaying backward) with your palm facing away from the body, *that means your halo is in the correct position and does not need to be flipped.* Any other combination — weak-strong, strong-strong, or weak-weak — means you need to flip that halo.

8. To energy test your root halo, follow the same procedure. Place one hand on your solar plexus and use the other to energy localize your root halo. Your palm facing your torso should test strong. Your palm facing away from your torso should test weak. Any other result means your root halo needs to be flipped.

9. To energy test your earth halo, use the option of imagining your arms are very long and reach down with your testing hand, miming the action of placing it on the earth halo, with your palm facing your body. Then test using your pendulum motion. Your palm facing the body should test strong, and the palm facing away should test weak. Any other result means your earth halo needs to be flipped.

10. To energy test your ming men halo, place your palm flat on the ming men if you can reach it and energy test. (If you can't reach it, then use the option of miming the action while focusing your intention on the ming men halo.) It should test strong when your palm is facing your body and weak when your palm is facing away. Any other combination means your ming men halo needs to be flipped.

Which Stream Do I Visit When?

Meridian Name	Stream	Cosmic Source	Element
Central	Conception	Earth herself and the air that buoys you	Air
Governing	Comprehension	Sky or soul's star	Air
Kidney	Waters of life	Waters	Water
Bladder	Distribution	Beauty through aura and senses	Water
Liver	Purpose	Shared root system	Wood
Gallbladder	Enactor/enforcer	Helmet of service	Wood
Triple Warmer	Energizer	Sunlight	Fire
Circulation/sex	Yin protector	Moon energy	Fire
Heart	Heart/connection	Heart of the Divine, earth, truth	Fire

Meridian Name	Stream	Cosmic Source	Element
Small intestine	Choice/ discernment	Web of connections	Fire
Spleen	Nourishment	Mother earth nourishment	Earth
Stomach	Embodiment	Collective experience	Earth
Lung	Give and receive	Enrichment from the world via the high heart	Metal
Large intestine	Distiller/refiner	Divine hook-up	Metal

ENERGETIC SPINE

Good for *grounding, rooting, centering,* and *anchoring.*

Conception (Central) Vessel and Comprehension (Governing) Vessel

The cosmic source of the conception vessel is the earth herself and the air surrounding her, which buoys you.

The cosmic source of the comprehension vessel is the sky — or you can use your soul's star (the star with your name on it) if you wish.

Although we usually trace them both upward from the root, in their circular microcosmic orbit, the conception corridor arises from the earth, and the comprehension corridor descends from the sky. The energies mix in their shared orbit, traveling in both directions.

You actually have three cosmic sources meeting in the energetic spine, since it is also the seat of the grid, whose cosmic source is the soul. These three cosmic sources — earth, sky, and the soul — source your three selves: Earth Elemental Self, Talking Self, and Wiser Self.

Conception vessel is the place where you take in energies and give birth both literally and figuratively to ideas, projects, knowing. This is the birthplace, the core, of your energies. It is a good place to visit when you want to investigate what is influencing you, from without and within. It is also a good place to plant affirmations and intentions. Any health issues affecting your midline can be explored here.

Comprehension vessel is the stream that connects most directly to your brain, so it is a great place to come when you need to formulate understanding or conscious awareness. But don't worry about getting clear, direct answers — just know that if you put in the request, your librarians will work on it in the background, until they can fulfill it. This is also a good stream to visit when you have physical issues with your spine or in your brain or with connecting brain and body. (For these types of issues you may also want to visit the distribution/bladder stream, which runs along the spine and governs the nervous system; see pages 227–28.)

WATER ELEMENT

Especially supports *resetting energy flow.*

Waters of Life Stream (Kidney Meridian; Yin Water)

The cosmic sources for this stream are the waters that renew and resuscitate the earth — moving underground, traveling over her surface, and existing within our environment.

The waters of life stream is the flow that brings in vital qi, or life force energy — the energy that feeds all the other streams. And its emotion is hope. Think of the phrase "Hope springs eternal." Its cosmic source is the waters of the earth, the springs, the damp, the rivers and lakes and oceans, the moisture patterns in weather, all moving in constant cycles of renewal.

This stream feeds your inner sense of knowing, your inner confidence and sense of self, and is also a wellspring of creativity. It is a place to come to just float and dream, to experience death and rebirth, or to close others out of the room so you can hear your own truth. It is a place to come to find balance — between yin and yang, between being and doing. To find renewal.

It is here that your being pulls in the vital energy to build bones, to create hormones, to fuel and nourish the operations of your Earth Elemental Self, to support your ability to hear, both literally and figuratively.

Distribution Stream (Bladder Meridian; Yang Water)

The cosmic source of this distribution stream filters into the body through your aura to enrich your senses. Reach out to gather in the beauty of sight and sound and sensation and fill your hands with this energy.

The distribution flow is also sometimes called the Guardian of the Peace, the Great Mediator, or the Minister of the Reservoir. It is charged with storing and distributing vital qi and fluid and eliminating excess energy and fluid. It communicates via your nervous system to sense what is needed, translate that into action, and integrate the operations of the body. It helps to regulate electrical communications in your body, alongside your heart/connection and comprehension streams.

This stream is a place to come to confront fear or when you feel dispirited, but it is also a place to visit when you feel hope rising and want to help yourself release the old and birth the new.

WOOD ELEMENT

Especially supports *coherence*: purpose and connectors.

Purpose Stream (Liver Meridian; Yin Wood)

Reach down into the shared root system beneath the earth to find the cosmic source of this stream.

Your purpose flow is a place to come when you need to support growth or address overgrowth of cells, thoughts, or behaviors in your body, mind, or spirit. It is a place to come to find your strength and your flexibility, your courage of conviction.

It is also a place to transform anger into purpose, frustration into a path forward. It is a place to come to support vision, both literal and figurative.

Enactor/Enforcer Stream
(Gallbladder Meridian; Yang Wood)

Access to the cosmic source comes through donning the helmet of service.

This stream is a good place to find your willingness to live your truth, to serve your truth. It is also a good place to let go of any feelings you might be holding on to: anger, resentment, emotions about past experiences, restlessness — everything that doesn't serve that truth in this moment.

This enactor/enforcer stream contains the energy that activates the unfolding of seeds: literal seeds and seed ideas, new paths, and new choices. If there are any decisions you are trying to make in your life or conflicts, double binds, or problems you are trying to resolve, let the spirits of this place speak to you. Ask for clarity, guidance, and practical suggestions.

FIRE ELEMENT

Especially supports *gatekeeping.*

Energizer Stream (Triple Warmer Meridian;
Yang Fire, Yang Gatekeeper)

The cosmic source of the energizer stream is the sunlight, the enlivening light that animates the life force and warms and illuminates all living beings.

The energizer stream is a place to visit when you need to find safety in your outer reality: your life, your actions, your world. It is also a place to come when you find yourself struggling with your identity in the world or in the eyes of others or when you want to address the various forms of yang gatekeeper reactivity: fight, flight, flood, flutter, fiddle.

The energizer stream helps you distribute vital qi: it is the stream to turn to when you want to manage stress hormones or immune system responses and mediate between water, or source qi, and fire, or gatekeeping qi.

It is a place to visit to meet with your energetic budget director: to allocate resources, fund certain choices, defund others. And where you can visit when habits keep you from enacting your heart's desire or conscious choice. Also a good place to drop into when dealing with physical immune system symptoms or sluggish immunity.

Yin Protector Stream
(Circulation/Sex Meridian; Yin Fire, Yin Gatekeeper)

The cosmic source of the yin protector stream is the moon, aligning you with the pull of the tides, the turning of cycles. It represents the inner knowing reflected in the outer world, as moonlight is a reflection of the sunlight. It illuminates the night, the unknowing, giving the gift of vision in the darkness.

The yin protector stream is a place to come to explore issues of self-protection, particularly relating to your inner sanctity of self, your inner identity. It is a place to come when your heart or inner core feel challenged, when you are reacting to situations with freeze, fog, fade, fatigue, faint, fall apart, fumble, falter, fail, or fibrillate. It is also a place to come when you need to open to others or let go and relax muscles in the body.

This stream is helpful when you have any challenges relating to self-regulation. The physical pathway associated with this stream is the vagus nerve. It is a place to visit when you want to address stage fright, fainting, digestion, reproductive hormones, blood circulation, or other regulation of fluids in your body.

Heart/Connection Stream (Heart Meridian; Yin Fire)

The cosmic source for the heart/connection stream is the heart of the Divine, heart of mother earth, or heart of truth.

This is the place to come to take refuge, to renew your allegiance to what you hold dear, to find sanctuary, to explore your feelings, to encounter your Wiser Self, and to listen to the dictates of your spirit.

Similarly, it is a place to visit when you are experiencing electrical disturbances (see also waters of life and distribution streams, since water conducts electricity through the body); issues with rhythm, pulse, blood circulation, or spirit; or fatigue, insomnia, dizziness, anxiety, love woes, stuttering, or mental imbalances.

Choice/Discernment Stream
(Small Intestine Meridian; Yang Fire)

The cosmic source for the choice/discernment stream is the web of connections, the swarm of all-knowing from which you choose and activate individual strands to create the story line of your life. Reach out to your air roots or down into your earth roots to access this source.

This is the stream to visit when you are trying to sort out your experience, when you have some choice you need to make or problem to solve, or when you are trying to find your own truth. This stream gives you access to your gut knowing.

The choice/discernment stream helps you to sort truth from untruth, pure from impure. It is a great place to visit when you are having trouble trusting your own judgment. It is also a place to visit when your digestion (literal or figurative) is challenged and you aren't gleaning the nutrients from your food or experiences.

Fire is about fueling action, so visits here can help you not only to choose but also to recognize concrete actions or steps you can take to set choices in motion.

EARTH ELEMENT

Especially supports *grounding, centering, rooting,* and *anchoring.*

Nourishment Stream (Spleen Meridian; Yin Earth)

The cosmic source for this stream is the universal flow from mother earth, a ceaseless energy of nourishment and caring.

This nourishment stream is your inner carer. It brings you the ability to extract nutrients from the earth; to help you metabolize food, experience, and feelings; and to use them to build or repair tissue, strengthen blood, renew cellular energy, and support healing.

This flow is often drained by the energizer stream, so it is important to support and reinforce this stream when stress has depleted you or you are dealing with autoimmune challenges. Metabolizing eights are especially helpful to support your nourishment stream.

Embodiment Stream (Stomach Meridian; Yang Earth)

The cosmic feed for this stream comes from the shared world, our collective experience, and it enters via your eyes and mouth and face.

The embodiment stream helps you to stomach what comes at you, accept change, cope with the world, work with transitions, respond to events and energies of the world, embody your own truth, adapt your sense of yourself, and evolve as needed. It helps you, as the poet T. S. Eliot wrote, "to prepare a face to meet the faces that you meet." The path of this stream always reminds me of those theater masks of joy and sorrow.

It is a good place to visit to explore digestion issues, both literal and figurative. It is also a good place from which to address challenges that affect your face, such as sinus congestion, and to work to calm sound sensitivity.

Embodiment energy is both strong and sensitive. It surrounds and embraces you, and when its flow is healthy, it can feel a bit protective or just warm and supportive.

METAL ELEMENT

Especially supports *coherence*: structure and integration.

Give and Receive Stream (Lung Meridian; Yin Metal)

The cosmic source for this stream comes into you by way of your heart chakra, which spirals out and pulls enrichment in from the world.

This stream is a place to come to give and receive: awareness, resources, faith, breath, or the life force that your spirit and body and mind need in order to be truly alive. It is also a place to let go of whatever does not serve you.

It's a good stream to visit if you have lung or breathing issues.

Distiller/Refiner Stream
(Large Intestine Meridian; Yang Metal)

Access the cosmic source for the distiller/refiner flow via your index (pointer) finger. Plug it into the heart of the Divine for a Divine hook-up.

Your head, your heart, and your gut form three brains that work together to keep your energies moving and coherent. Your gut separates the food and energies you have digested into nutrients and refuse. It releases what your body cannot use and creates over thirty energetic messengers, neurotransmitters that regulate the workings of your head and heart and body. It is the place where what you take in from the world is distilled and transformed to serve your body, mind, and spirit.

This stream is a wonderful place to come to sort out your experiences and understand what you can use and what should be released. It is a place to come to transform painful or positive experience into understanding. It is a place to visit to learn lessons and then distill out principles, guidelines, and concepts to inform your future choices.

This energetic stream is intimately bound with the swarm of interconnections, with the root systems and mycelium and web of connections that link all of creation. The cells here respond not just to your own body's needs but to the collective consciousness of the microorganisms that live in your gut and in the earth, as well as to the shared consciousness.

⌾ Appendix C ⌾

List of Exercises, Protocols, and Guided Visits

Exercises and Protocols

Guided Visits

Notes

CHAPTER TWO: RENAME, REFRAME, AND RECLAIM

p. 29   *"What is cancer, ultimately?"*: Zach Bush, "Eat Dirt! And Thrive," lecture presented by PRFCT Earth Project, 1:30:33, YouTube, July 10, 2018, https://youtu.be/HL6OPzQe9Is.

CHAPTER THREE: JUST CONNECT

p. 49   *"Well, your toe bone"*: Will Osborne and Dick Rogers, "Dry Bones" (New York: Leeds Music Corp., 1940).

CHAPTER FOUR: BEYOND BINARY

p. 77   *In parts of Africa*: I first encountered this concept in conversations with Dr. J. L. Evans, director of the Consultative Group on Early Childhood Care and Development, whose work was based on cross-cultural child-rearing studies in developing countries from the 1960s through '90s. For a more contemporary (nonacademic) discussion, see Kelly Oakes, "Is the Western Way of Raising Kids Weird?," BBC Future, February 22, 2021, https://www.bbc.com/future/article/20210222-the-unusual-ways-western-parents-raise-children.

p. 84   *Have you seen: Fantastic Fungi*, directed by Louie Schwartzberg, written by Mark Monroe (Lake Oswego, OR: Area 23A, 2019), https://fantasticfungi.com.

CHAPTER FIVE: KEEPING THE GATES OF SELF

p. 95   *four major tasks*: If you are familiar with Donna Eden's work, you will recognize this as very similar to the Triple Warmer energy system. I wrote about the gatekeeper in my book *Listening In: Dialogues with the Wiser Self* in 1990 and was stunned to encounter such a similar explanation when I studied with Donna Eden nearly twenty years later.

p. 100   *She was strolling down a street*: Story retold with permission of Donna Eden. Her groundbreaking book *Energy Medicine* is a treasure trove of energy insights and energy medicine techniques. Donna Eden with David Feinstein, *Energy Medicine: Balancing Your Body's Energies for Optimal Health, Joy, and Vitality* (New York: Tarcher, 1998; New York: Penguin, 2008).

CHAPTER TWELVE: YOUR WEB OF MEANING

p. 243   *"Tracing Meridians with Donna Eden" video on YouTube*: Filmed by HipChicksCreate, 7:35, YouTube, September 28, 2017, https://www.youtube.com/watch?v=Vv5dkvMg1z4, or learn tracing meridians from any Eden Energy Medicine practitioner.

CHAPTER THIRTEEN: THE WEB OF CONNECTIONS

p. 257   *We used a version*: "Renovating the Rooms of Your Chakras" is a simplified version of a longer method I teach called "Storyline Track and Balance." A full class on this technique is available on DVD via my website, https://www.ellenmeredith.com.

p. 266   *I subsequently discovered*: Thanks to Doug J. Moore for helping locate a few of these sonar rings as I was developing this technique.

CHAPTER FOURTEEN: SPIRIT IN THE BODY

p. 283   *Figure-eight between your fully realized self*: You might be feeling a bit befuddled by all these "selves." Your Earth Elemental Self, Talking Self, and Wiser Self are three densities of your being. They work as a committee to create the person you know as "you." The harmonic self and fully realized selves are both templates set up to guide your gatekeeper in keeping you in form. Your harmonic self is a master template of identity you create with some input from your Wiser Self, based on your experiences and beliefs about who you are. Your fully realized self is a master template created by your soul and Wiser Self as a model of your truest potential. When we open the gates between these templates, we have clearer access to radiance and support to shift forms that don't represent our most fully realized expression of self.

Acknowledgments

In some ways, this book was written across lifetimes. And for that, I want to acknowledge my inner teachers — my Councils — who taught me how to listen and how to hear in the language of energy. And because they had so very much work to do to help me inhabit this body, this life, this story line, over the many years they've trained me, they get extra credit!

When I began to write *Your Body Will Show You the Way*, I was not sure what the way would be. My Councils said, "Change will be so rapid, you will need to write it for at least two years ahead of what you understand." I didn't quite know what they meant. And then, a few months later, we went on Covid-19 lockdown, and I realized that we had entered some kind of wormhole and that instead of just focusing on how to change the world, we would also need to learn how to navigate this world changing us.

And I am awed by the grace and flexibility with which many people did adjust to new reality after new reality. I want to acknowledge all those who stepped up to help other people, to enrich the web with creativity and cultural contributions, to the entertainers who learned to do their work differently, and of course to those frontline workers who didn't have the luxury of hiding out and wearing pajamas all day and fermenting

318

vegetables and Zooming to work. Thanks to them, we got groceries, and veterinary services, and health advice, and more toilet paper than we knew what to do with.

I want to acknowledge my very skillful agent, Steve Harris, who got my book where it belongs, and my wonderful publishers, New World Library, who launched my previous book at the beginning of the Covid-19 lockdown and have ushered this manuscript through its prepublication paces — still contending with Covid-19 restrictions — with skill and good humor. In particular, thanks to my editors Georgia Hughes, Kristen Cashman, and Diana Rico; proofreader Tanya Fox; designers Tona Pearce Myers, Tracy Cunningham, and Victoria Kuskowski; and of course my fabulous guide to getting this book out into view, Kim Corbin. Thanks also to all the people behind the scenes at NWL who have made production on this book as enjoyable as the last one.

This book is about learning to live from the inside out, finding inner teachers and positive outer teachers, and letting yourself be guided via your body. Ironically, I had a lot of outer teachers along the way who woke me up to this path: of course, Donna Eden goes to the head of the list, because she's such a trailblazer and wakes me up with every interaction. In the Eden world I want to also thank all my Eden Energy Medicine colleagues and buddies who helped me see how my inside-out training and many years of getting to know energy on the job could mesh with such a marvelous healing modality. Special shout-outs to Lauren Walker for her generous foreword, Paulette Taschereau, Douglas J. Moore, Susan Stone, Jeff Harris, Sara Allen, Sarah Buck, Stephanie Eldringhoff, Sandy Wand, Debra Hurt, Melanie Smith, and Madison King.

And I have to thank my wonderful students and clients, who taught me, through their stories and experiences and efforts, what it takes to heal and how to support that process.

Just as our outer world began to shut down, I was thrilled to be invited to join the Shift Network faculty and bring my teaching online. Special thanks to Nick Mattos, CarolAnne Robinson, hosts Hiroki and Lauren, and all the wonderful staff who walk their talk; the great students from around the globe; and my TAs, Stacy Newman, Shura Gat, and Julie Fowler. Check out my courses there (theshiftnetwork.com/faculty), available on demand for streaming in this new, crazy web world. It was such fun to bring this material alive and field-test it with real people in real and virtually real time!

Beyond that, I want to thank Sandy Boucher for a great story she loaned me; Richard Lalli, who can always get me to laugh and lighten up; Kendra Barron for her artistry; Dave Weikart for introducing me to learning from the inside out; Marty and Bonnie for stepping in as a team to help Mom transition; Barbara Allen, DC, for giving me a workplace to learn my craft; Ruth Denison for teaching me about breathing and walking; Diane Vreuls and Stuart Friebert, my first writing teachers; Irene Young, photographer extraordinaire; and Lee Harris and Kim Seer for their contributions to my understanding of the unseen worlds.

And always, I am grateful to Judith, my partner of thirty-five years, for her quiet strength, and to my cats and dogs, who kept me sane when this earth dimension seemed so alien to me.

If I didn't mention you by name, please know that everyone I've met in this life, and who echoed through to me from other lives, has contributed to the web of meaning I feel blessed to present in this book.

Index

Page references followed by an italicized *fig.* indicate illustrations. Page references followed by an italicized *t.* indicate tables. When multiple references for exercises or protocols are given, page references in **bold** indicate instructions for how to perform the exercise.

inner guidance: author's experience,
1–4, 12, 118–21; energy medicine
and, 4–5; faulty grounding and, 148;
gatekeeper as conduit of, 94–95;
inside-out thinking and, 13–15;
reclaiming, 39–40
inner structures, 250, 311
inner teachers, 40, 118–21. *See also*
Councils
inner wisdom, 5; access to, 292; exercises/
protocols, 290–91; grounding in, 159,
160 (*see also* grounding); outside-in
thinking and, 160. *See also* spiritual
wisdom
inside-out thinking: anchoring, 165;
author's experience, 11–12; character-
istics of, 13; connection and, 62–64;
disease/illness and, 18–20; during
empowered yin era, 12–13; interpreting experience with, 299; outside-in
thinking vs., 13–17, 23–25; Play with
It!, 17; purpose and, 186; spiritual
wisdom and, 286; transforming to,
25–26; web of connections and, 19
insomnia, 198
integrations, 181, 201–3, 262 *fig. 13.1*, 299,
311
intention, 47, 122, 200
inter-connection: blindness to, 247;
coincidences and, 255; Covid-19
pandemic and, 83; distiller/refiner
stream and, 208, 312; gatekeeper and,
95; healing and, 51; in nature, 84, 247;
self/world exchange and, 255; spheric
consciousness rooted in, 87–88, 122;
web of connections and, 247; yang
view of, 84–85; yin view of, 19. *See
also* web of connections
internet, 248
intestines, 295–96
intuition, 240, 243, 261
irritable bowel syndrome (IBS), 198
isolation, 50

journaling, 41, 164, 290
judgment, 38
Just Connect (protocol), 51–54, 52 *fig. 3.1*

Kabbalah, 80
keyed containers, 252
Kidney-1 points, 114, 115 *fig. 5.8*, 217, 224,
224 *fig. 11.2*
Kidney-10 points, 114, 115 *fig. 5.8*
Kidney-27 points, 115 *fig. 5.8*, 116, 225,
226, 301
kidney meridian, 224–25, 224 *figs.
11.2–11.3*, 304 *t.*, 306–7. *See also* waters
of life stream
kindness, 221
knee boxes, 66, 67–68
knees, 269 *t. 1*
knowledge, 225

language of energy: body/mind/spirit
and, 8; dialogue with body and, 32;
energy medicine and, 4–5; learning
to speak, 9, 25–26, 40; outside-in
thinking and, 245; syntax of, 26; vocabulary of, 244; web of connections
and, 26
Language Your Body Speaks, The
(Meredith), 40, 102, 147, 237
large intestine meridian, 207 *fig. 10.4*,
305 *t.*, 311–12. *See also* distiller/refiner
stream
larger mind / smaller mind concept,
287–89
Let the Earth Breathe You (exercise), 78
life flow, 219–20
life force, 205
life-forms, 71; communication with
83–84, 189; web of, 247
lifestyle, 2
lifestyle medicine, 9, 219–20
light, 270 *t. 1*; circulation of, 216–17
Listening In (Meredith), 316n1 (ch. 5)
lived experience, 15–16

About the Author

Ellen Meredith, Doctor of Arts, is a conscious channel, medical intuitive, energy medicine practitioner, teacher, writer, traveler, framer, messenger, and visionary. She has been in practice since 1984, helping over ten thousand clients and students across the globe tune in to and communicate with their own energies, hear their inner guidance, and heal.

Ellen is renowned for her down-to-earth yet out-of-the-box thinking. Her approach to self-healing with energy medicine offers readers ways to understand and get to the heart of their health and life challenges and to work compassionately with their body, mind, and spiritual dimensions.

She builds on everyday experiences and commonsense frameworks, believing that life reveals more of its meaning if you treat it as an evolving story and see yourself as a unique character helping to co-create it.

Originally trained as a healer by her inner teachers (Councils), Ellen later became an Eden Energy Medicine Advanced Practitioner (EEMAP), served on Donna Eden's faculty, and joined the faculty of the Shift Network, where she offers online courses and can be found presenting on multiple online summits. She brings humanity, humor, and insight in many forms to the world of energy healing.

Ellen is the author of *The Language Your Body Speaks: Self-Healing with Energy Medicine* (New World Library, 2020), *Listening In: Dialogues with the Wiser Self*, the audiobook *In Search of Radiance: Learning to Stand with Your Wiser Self*, and numerous video classes on energy medicine, including "Energy Fluency," "Gatekeeper," "Energy Chiro," "Storyline Track and Balance," "Energy Wisdom," "Intuition and Practitioner's Mind," and "Healing Spaces." Using the name Ellen M. Ilfeld, she has also published several books on child development, including *Learning Comes to Life: An Active Learning Program for Teens, Good Beginnings: Parenting in the Early Years,* and *Early Childhood Counts: A Programming Guide on Early Childhood Care for Development.*

Learn more at ellenmeredith.com.